THE LADY IS A VETERINARIAN

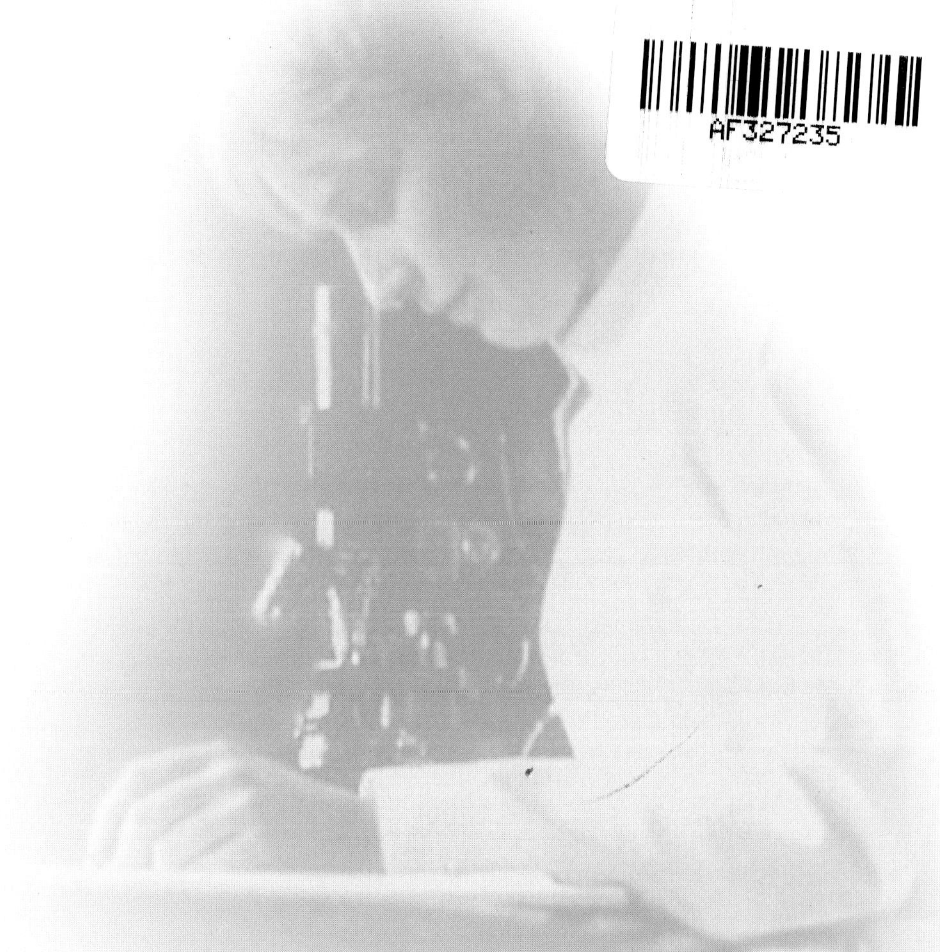

The Pioneer Women Who Graduated from
The School of Veterinary Medicine, Kansas State College
1932–1956

Lesley Ann Gentry

THE LADY IS A VETERINARIAN

Library of Congress Control Number: 2005927737
ISBN Number: 0-9767871-0-5

Graphic Design & Book layout by Larry G. Nichols II
Printed in the U.S.A. by Mennonite Press, Inc., Newton, KS
        First Printing June, 2005.

Gentry, Lesley A.
The Lady Is A Veterinarian
1. History, Kansas, Veterinary Medicine, Womens Historical Study

To all my family here, there and in my heart.

Acknowledgements

*S*o many people have helped me with this book that it is impossible for me to mention them all. I have been blessed with help from wonderful people here in the USA, and good folks in the UK.

My first thank you must be for Dr. Phyllis (Hickney) Larsen, who has inspired me to do so much more than I ever thought I could. I have learned so much from you about women in veterinary medicine. You truly have been a great mentor to me!

Invaluable help and information came from many resources; special thanks to Myrna Gleue, at Kansas State University, who in the early days of my research helped so much. I greatly appreciated all the help of Dr's Elmore and Erickson, Cheri Ubel and Pat Patton at Kansas State University gave me. A special thank you to Dr. Peter Chenoweth for his friendship and support of my book.

I always appreciated the invaluable information and kind help that Diane Fagen, at the AVMA library gave me.

I am indebted to the families and friends of these women, for supplying me with information, articles and photos.

I wish to thank my husband and children for being so tolerant of me when I thought I did not know what I was doing! I appreciate so much, the editing on the book that my daughter Jamie has done for me.

Finally, a big thank you to Cary Christensen, DVM, Director of Strategic Development and Veterinary Services, at Bayer Healthcare, LLC. for his support of this book. It is with the help of Dr. Christensen, and Dr. Lynn Allen, Director of Veterinary Services. at Bayer Healthcare, LLC, that I proudly have Bayer as sponsor of this book.

— Lesley Ann Gentry

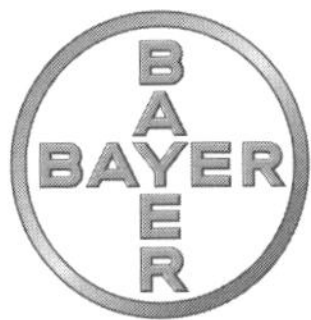

Bayer HealthCare

Foreword

"All of us are but his instruments, who do our little bit and pass by."
— Mother Teresa

My father Alfred Wight – better known to his millions of readers as author and veterinarian James Herriot – was one of the most appreciative men I have known. Being such an astute observer of human nature, he could appreciate qualities in others, good and bad.

My father had a deep respect for the 'fairer' sex, and considered that hard physical labour was never a 'job for a woman.' I think it was a combination of seeing the slavish daily grind for the farmers' wives, as well as my mother's dogged cleaning and scrubbing of the long stone passageways of our home, the big rambling 'Skeldale House,' that was responsible for his determination to dissuade my sister, Rosie, from becoming a veterinarian.

'Don't be a vet Rosie,' he used to say. 'It is a rough job and no job for a woman!'

In his day, of course, the standing of the female in society was on a vastly different plane to what it is today. Positions of authority – especially among the professional classes – were overwhelmingly occupied by men. Nowhere was this more graphically illustrated than in the Veterinary Profession. A female veterinarian was a rare sight indeed.

In my father's first year at Glasgow Veterinary College in 1933 there was in his words, 'one solitary frightened looking little girl'. When I entered Glasgow veterinary School almost thirty years later, there were only six women in a class of forty six veterinary undergraduates, but in 1998, while attending the graduation in Glasgow for the veterinary faculty, I noticed that over seventy five percent of the fresh-faced young veterinary surgeons were women!

In 1980, in our practice here in Thirsk, we employed our first female veterinary assistant. This was a milestone, as it was almost unheard of to employ a female for the rough and tumble of large animal practice in Yorkshire. One of my father's best friends, Basil Aylward who ran the veterinary practice in nearby Richmond in the Yorkshire dales, married a veterinary surgeon, and Kate Aylward continued to work very successfully for many years among the

Dales farmers. My father used to say to me 'You know, Kate copes very well among the farmers up there! She is actually very popular!'

He still clung to the old fashioned belief that a country vet's work was really for a man, but his opinion was steered in another direction after employing our first female vet, as she not only performed the work assigned to her to a very high standard, but gained the respect and admiration of our own farmer clients.

I remember I had the drop on her only once. She rang for assistance one evening for help with a particularly difficult calving, where the calf was presented with its head turned back in the womb... In a case such as this, where every extra inch of reach can be vital, I have always stripped to the waist to allow maximum arm length while trying to grasp the tantalizingly, and just 'out-of-reach,' nose of the calf.

'I would strip off to the waist if I were you, Jane!' I said to her. 'Getting rid of that cumbersome parturition overall will give you that little bit of extra reach which will probably enable you to reach the calf's head.'

Being a modest young lady, she refused to do this, despite calls of encouragement from the farmers. 'We don't mind, Jane! Don't bother about us!'

She still refused so, to the farm lads' obvious disappointment, it was I who had to strip off and do the job for her. From that day on, she wore a short-sleeved vest to every calving case.

On another occasion I found that I had something to learn from her. She had performed a caesarian section on a cow that, due to no fault of hers, died a few days later. The following week, I performed a caesarian on the same farm with a satisfying outcome. One of the farmer workers who had assisted on both the operations was a friend of mine, and we were walking in the hills of Lake District one day when he suddenly said, 'That young girl vet you 'ave now, by… she is a good vet! I 'ave nothing but admiration for 'er. She never gave up on that job; never knew when she were beaten! She did a marvelous job!'

I stayed silent, as there was no praise forthcoming for my operation, one that had resulted in a healthy mother and a fine young calf.

There were a few moments' silence before he spoke again. 'An a'll tell yer summat else!' he continued. 'There was none o' that cussin' and swearin' that went on when you did yours!'

Perhaps the young 'lady vet' had something to teach me about the 'art' of veterinary practice, as well as the 'science.'

James Herriot and his partner Siegfred could see, all those years ago, the vast changes that would blanket their profession, but neither of them could have foreseen one of its most remarkable transformations, the steadily progressive integration of women into a field of endeavor that, just thirty years ago, was regarded as a predominantly a male domain. Not only have they established themselves in positions of authority within all branches of veterinary work, but they have demonstrated that they are more than capable of making every bit a good a job of it as their male counterparts have done in the past.

As veterinarians, we are privileged to be part of a profession that has rich and varied history, and Lesley's book about the pioneering days of women within our profession, illustrates the early beginnings of one of its most dramatic metamorphoses.

In my tours of the country, speaking about my life as a vet and that of my father, I am often approached for advice by young girls who wish to become veterinarians.

I invariably reply, 'Go for it! It is a great profession and you girls are now very much part of its future!' I have no doubt that the face of the profession will see yet more changes in the years to come but, in this respect, it may well be that it will alter very little.

— Jim Wight, M.R.C.V.S

Introduction

In the year 1897 William Augustine Byrne, (veterinarian) in speaking to the Irish Central Veterinary Society, mentioned in a paper he read on Veterinary Ethics that "Women will, of course, be admitted to the veterinary profession." He would later follow through with this remark to have as an assistant, Aleen Cust Britain's first woman veterinarian.

Aleen would be followed by many women from around the world in her chosen profession. Some of the early women who came to follow Aleen, I am proud to boast, would be from Kansas State College, Division of Veterinary Medicine.

Helen Richt, 1932, and Louise Sklar, 1934, both determined and courageous women, who dared to challenge a profession that was not considered a place for *ladies*, were the first two to graduate. Kansas State College was most gracious to minorities of which these women were included.

The twelve women I have chosen to write about from 1932 - 1956 probably had to overcome the biggest hurdles, not that they felt challenged by this idea. These women, all diverse in character, enjoyed their work, all having a passionate interest in the animals in their care.

They, along with all the incredible women who followed them, have paved a better future, for the women veterinarians of today!

Table of Contents

Chapter 1

Helen S. Richt
–1932 Division of Veterinary Medicine
Kansas State College

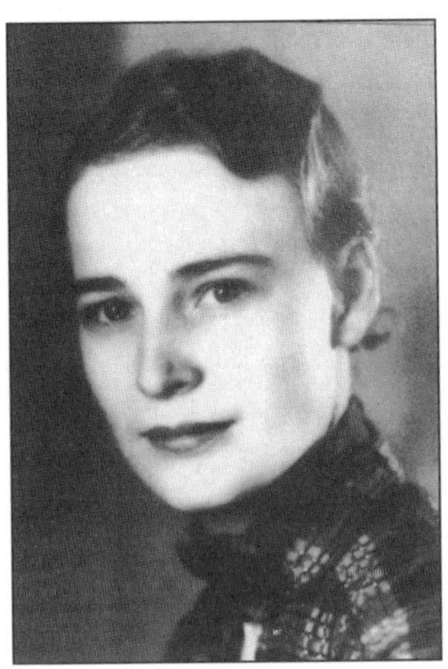

Helen Sophie Richt was born October 9, 1910 to William J. Richt and Elizabeth "Bowley" Richt, in Sarpy County, Omaha, Nebraska. She was the fourth of eleven children born to this union.

Helen was a happy child and enjoyed her sisters Florence, Ethel, Hazel, Pearl, Ruth, Edith and Alice and brothers William, Jack and the youngest of the Richt family, Dick.

The Richt children all attended the public school system in Omaha.

The family farm was a haven for the children, especially Helen. She loved all the farm animals but had a passion for the dogs and cats.

Helen who was known as 'Sis' to her family, was a determined, strong-willed young girl. Her sister Edith described Helen as being an 'out-doorsy' sort of a girl, but not a tomboy!

It was not sure when, but it was obvious from a very young age that Helen loved animals, and showed a great desire to take care of them.

Whilst Helen's loving mother Elizabeth was taking care of the Richt house

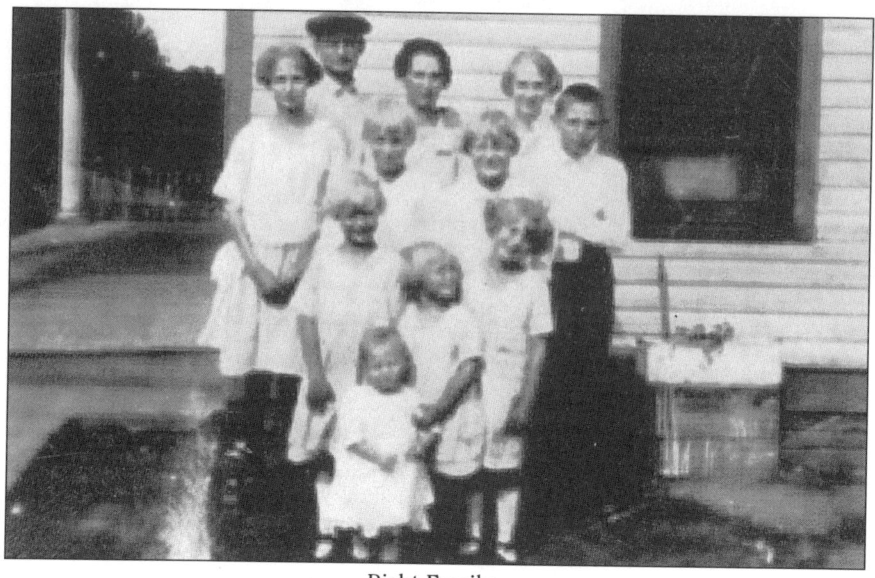

Richt Family

hold, her father was busy taking care of the family farm and also working at a serum company in Omaha.

Helen's father was a hardworking, knowledgeable man who enjoyed his family and neighbors. The way in which he cared for animals on their farm left a great impression on young Helen. She was her father's shadow, spending a great deal of time following and helping him.

Helen's youngest brother Dick remembers that their father was considered an 'unlicensed country vet,' always helping take care of the animals in the neighborhood. Subsequently, inspiring the animal loving Helen!

Another inspiration to Helen was Dr. Don W. Walker, a 1918 graduate of the Kansas City Veterinary College.

Dr. Walker, a good friend of the family, was also a partner with Helen's father in a feedlot operation they had at their farm.

If Helen was not helping Dr. Walker or her father with the farm animals, she might be found reading. What Helen could not learn about animals from the men, she gained knowledge about from books. Helen loved to read and when her mother needed her to take care of more domestic duties; she could be found hiding in the outhouse reading!

As Helen approached her graduation from high school her desire to work with animals was greater than ever. Her father encouraged her in her desire, knowing that this was a profession that was 'male dominated' and that Helen would have much to contend with.

And so it was, with Helen's excellent grades and the support and encouragement of her father and Dr. Walker, Helen applied to veterinary school at Kansas State College.

Upon Helen's graduation from South Omaha High School in Omaha, Nebraska in the summer of 1928, she was delighted to find out that she had been accepted to veterinary school.

It was not enough to find out that her childhood dream had come to fruition, but also that she was the *first female* ever to be accepted to the veterinary professional curriculum at Kansas State College!

The first day of veterinary school for Helen was not only a memorable one for her, but a momentous occasion for Kansas State College.

For the attractive young Helen, each day was a new challenge. She stayed focused on her classes and ignored the disparaging remarks when she could. Maybe it was her German ancestry that kept her 'strong.' Helen took it all in her stride.

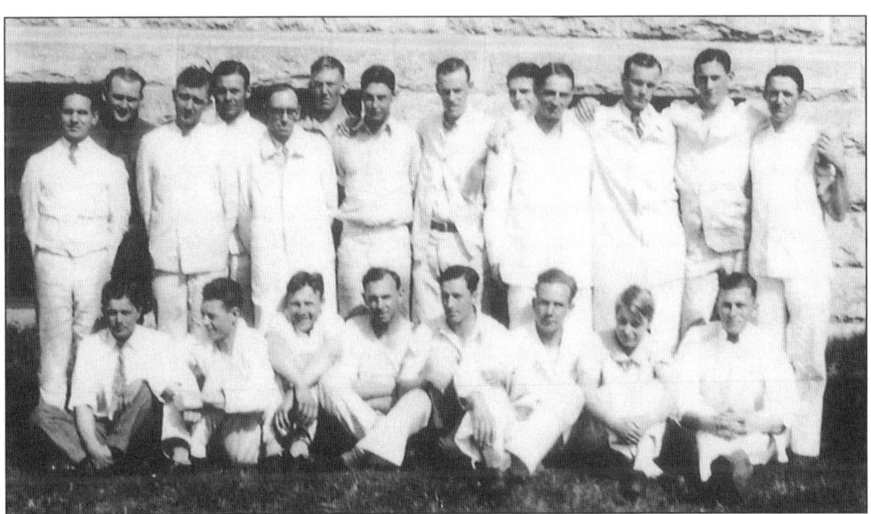

Helen and her classmates, circa 1931

Helen enjoyed her classes, learning as much as she could. At times she was astonished at the attention she drew as being the 'first woman' in veterinary school at Kansas State. To Helen it was no big thing; after all she was there because she loved animals.

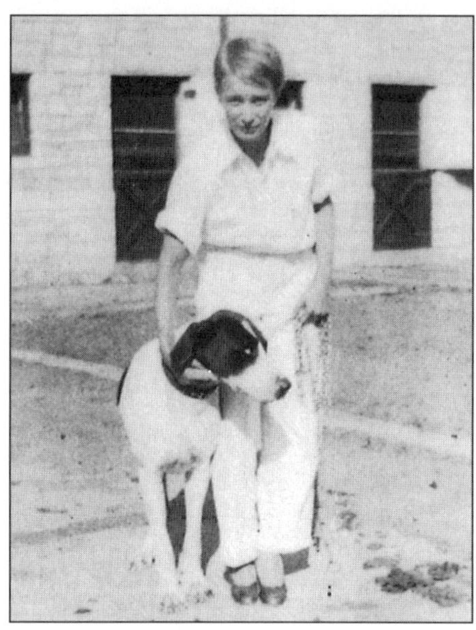
Helen as a student, circa 1930

The newspapers saw it differently though and sought her out when they could for a story. The reporters knew that Helen was not just a first to Kansas State, but would be included in the first thirty women veterinarians in the country!

A particularly nice article about Helen was featured in the February 1929 issue of *The Jen-Sal Journal*. A photograph of Helen sitting at a microscope (on the cover of this book) clearly showed a dedicated woman.

Helen's outgoing personality kept her in good stead and she had no problems making new friends. She was active in the Women's Athletic Association, and enjoyed playing baseball, volleyball and hockey.

Helen was also a junior member of the Kansas State Chapter of the American Veterinary Medical Association. The chapter having only been formed two years earlier helped students to promote interest and activity in the study of Veterinary medicine.

After completing approximately one hundred and sixty - four credit hours, Helen graduated with her degree, Doctor of Veterinary Medicine, on June 2, 1932, alongside eighteen men.

Helen was also honored with the Franklin Prize in Pathology. The donor of the ten dollar first place prize was O. M. Franklin, a graduate of Kansas State College, Division of Veterinary Medicine in 1912.

Dr. Helen Richt was recorded as taking her Kansas State Board exams on May 24, 1932. She was the first female to come before the examining board. Dr A. F. Wempe, chairman of the examining board, was noted as saying that Helen had submitted excellent papers. Helen was pleased to receive an excellent grade, which was considerably higher than some of her male counterparts recorded at this time!

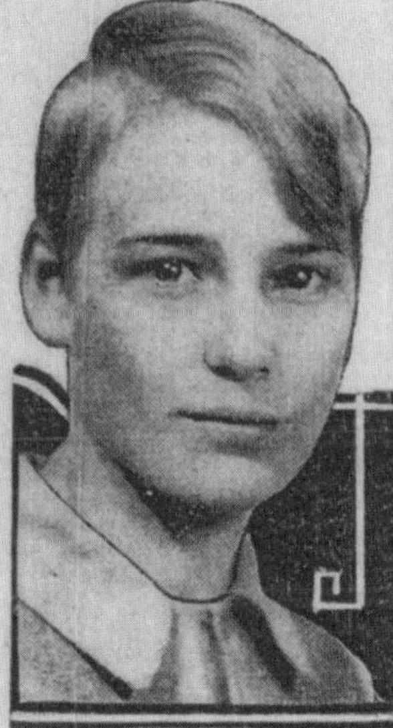

Omaha Girl Is First to Appear Before Kansas Veterinary Board

For the first time in Kansas history a woman appeared before the Kansas board of veterinarian examiners Tuesday seeking a certificate to practice "animal doctoring" in the state.

She was Miss Helen Richt of Omaha, pretty 21-year-old student at Kansas State college, one of 20 to take the board's spring examination, says an Associated Press dispatch. Miss Richt is to receive her degree of veterinary medicine at the college this spring after four years' work.

Miss Richt, the dispatch added, said she did not know where she would locate but was most interested in small animal and laboratory work. Her professors at the college said she had skillfully handled all laboratory work while at school except that she did not work on "large animal" cases.

She is a daughter of Mr. and Mrs. William Richt, Route 3, South Omaha. She was graduated from South High in 1928.

A love of pets and a desire to establish a hospital for their care led her to take up the study, she says.

Helen Richt.

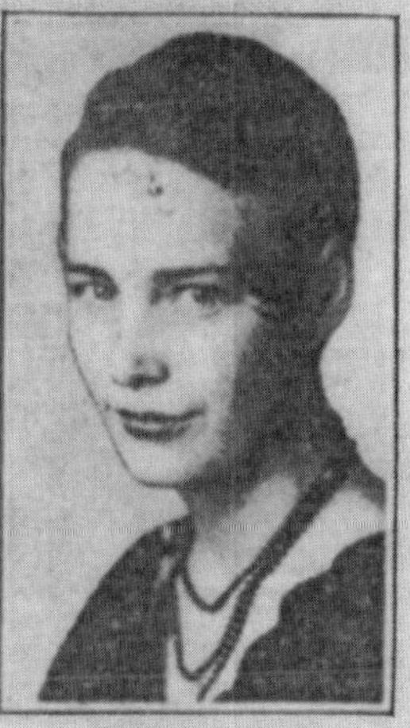

Graduate Veterinarian

Miss Helen Richt.

Nebraska Girl Pioneers at Kansas State College.

Miss Helen Richt, 21 years old, is the first woman to enroll and be graduated from Kansas State college in the curriculum of veterinary medicine. She lives in South Omaha, Neb. Four years ago Miss Richt went to K. S. C. as a retiring freshman coed—she didn't much like the publicity given her as the only woman veterinary medicine student but she got a lot of attention nevertheless. She said then that she was especially interested in small animal hospital work and she plans to do that sort of work after graduation.

Her instructors say Miss Richt has been a good student and has done all the undergraduate work required. She recently passed the examination before the state veterinary board, the first woman ever to be examined.

Helen did not forget her family back in Omaha, and enjoyed visiting the family when she could. On one of her visits home, her younger brother Jack remembers his sister Dr. Helen taking care of one of the family's pets. It happened that a German Shepherd pup that the family had raised had caught his leg in a fence. After Helen had examined the badly injured leg it was determined that the leg would need to be amputated. Helen instructed her father to gather a list of supplies from Dr. Walker. On preparing the animal on a table in the house, Helen performed the necessary surgery. The pup recovered and later was placed with friends of the family and did just fine. Jack was so proud to watch his big sister perform surgery!

For the 1933 -1934 school year Helen was engaged as a technician in the Pathology laboratory at the veterinary division.

It was during this time that she met and courted a handsome veterinary student by the name of William "Bill" Irwin. Bill graduated with the class of 1933.

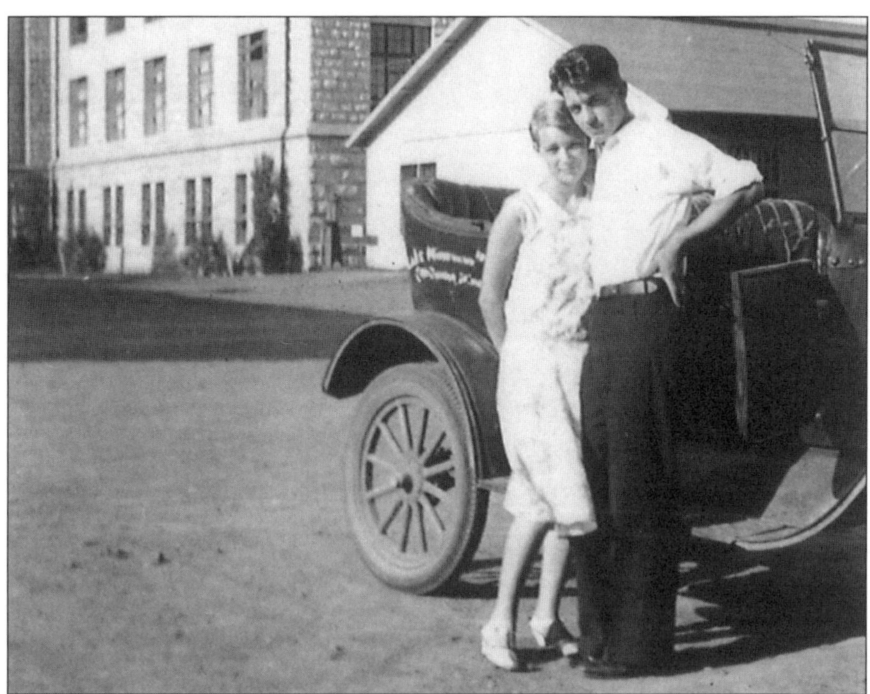

Bill and Helen in Manhattan, Kansas, circa 1933

Helen was proud to join the faculty at the veterinary division for the school year 1934 -1935 school year. It was an honor for her to work with Dean Dykstra, a man who was considered to be a very fair gentleman!

It was also good to have another female, Dr. Louise Sklar, who had graduated with the class of 1934, to confer with.

Helen did take time out of her Christmas vacation to marry Bill. Dr's Irwin and Richt were united in marriage December 30, 1934.

Dr. Bill Irwin worked for the next year, 1935, for the US Government, testing cattle for Bangs (Brucellosis.)

It was in 1935 that it came to Bill and Helen's attention of a practice in Tulsa, Oklahoma, that was for sale. The owner of the practice, a Dr. Walter's, had recently passed away. Bill and Helen were happy to purchase the practice 'The City Veterinary Hospital.' They rented the buildings and the lower level of the house that Mrs. Walter owned. The house was on the same lot on Sixth and Madison Street as the veterinary hospital.

Bill and Helen enjoyed working together at the hospital. Helen performed tonsillectomies and caesareans, taking great care to make sure her patients were comfortable. She was good at calming stressed animals, not afraid to handle the biggest of dogs. There was no doubt that she was a 'gutsy' lady!

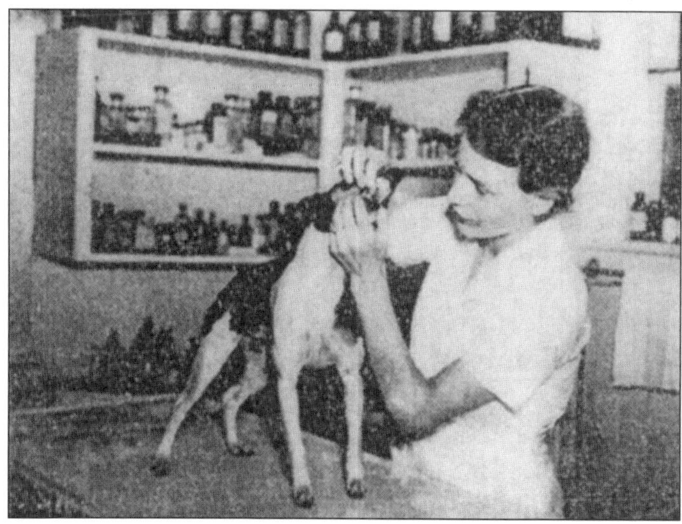

Helen examining a patient, circa 1935

Helen was in her element, after all, this had been her dream. She was a loving and compassionate veterinarian, appreciated not only by the animals but by their owner's too.

The Irwin's enjoyed several of their own dogs, their favorite two probably being 'Billy,' an English Setter, and 'Fritz,' a Schnauzer. No doubt, they were two well cared for dogs with two vets in the house!

Helen was noted as saying to a reporter in regards to her work, "It is hard work, but there is a lot of satisfaction in helping some poor dog or cat. It's a matter of loving animals. I've always been interested in taking care of unfortunate creatures."

In the spring of 1937, Bill and Helen were made happy by the birth of their firstborn, a son William, born on the 24th of April. Helen spent less time at the hospital, staying home to care for baby William.

The year could not have been more joyous when Dr. Helen "Richt" Irwin was appointed Secretary of the Section on Small Animals. She was the first woman veterinarian to hold an office in the American Veterinary Medical Association! This was a tremendous accomplishment in 1937 when the field of small animals was still finding its place in the veterinary world.

Helen and Bill were blessed with a second son Tom, born on April 17, 1940.

Helen and her husband had worked hard in their practice, establishing a good clientele. They were excited when they built a beautiful new small animal hospital at Thirty Sixth Street and Peoria in South Tulsa, in 1942. The Art Deco building was registered on the National Register of Art Deco Places. Tulsa is well known for this type of architecture. In 1945, the new 'City Veterinary Hospital' was considered to be one of America's model small animal hospitals!

Bill and Helen enjoyed having Loyd Irwin, one of Bill's younger brother's, work for them as 'night man' in the hospital. Loyd slept at the hospital and watched over the animals.

After moving to Oklahoma, Helen and Bill stayed loyal to their Alma Mater by attending meetings and sending contributions for the Reading Room (Library) at the veterinary school. Helen and Bill were observed taking a constructive part in the Kansas Veterinary Medical Associations State meeting in Wichita, Kansas in January of 1942.

Helen helped Bill in the hospital when she could, but retired from active practice after the birth of their third son Patrick, on November 11, 1945. She was kept busy with their three boys. In referring to a newspaper article written about Helen and her handling a dog, her youngest son Pat confers that "she was pretty darn good with kids too!"

Even though Helen did not stay in active practice, she endeavored to do her part for veterinary medicine. In 1955, she served as Secretary to the Oklahoma Veterinary Medical Association's Auxiliary.

Helen kept up with veterinary medicine by reading journals and accompanying her husband Bill all over the country to many meetings. Bill was an accomplished speaker, presenting many speeches on small animal practice. Helen was proud to be with Bill when he spoke to the Junior Chapter of the American Veterinary Medical Association in Manhattan, in the early 1950's. Often times, they were happy to have their dear friends Dr. E. R. Walker, another veterinarian, and his wife Jeanie from Pawhuska, Oklahoma, ride along with them.

Helen's son Tom remembers his mother and father working as a team, and that his dad never made a decision without Helen's input. He remembers that when his father returned home from the hospital in the evening, he would sit and discuss cases with Helen, appreciating her opinion.

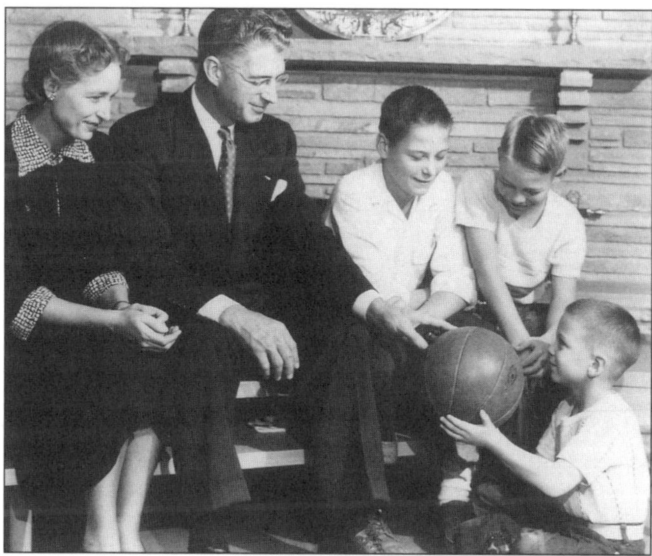

The Richt Family

Bill obviously held his wife in high regard, honoring her by keeping her name on the roster of veterinarians on the front door of the hospital.

On September 10, 1959, a shadow cast itself over the Irwin home. Bill, who had been on a hunting trip in Alaska, was killed in a tragic airplane accident. One of America's outstanding practitioners was gone. Helen and the boys were devastated.

Helen sold their beloved 'City Veterinary Hospital' to a veterinarian that she and Bill had known. With sons William and Tom away at college, Helen was thankful to members of family on both sides for rallying to help her and young Patrick who was still at home.

Moving on, as she knew Bill would want her to do, Helen who was still active in the Oklahoma Veterinary Association was elected as Treasurer in 1960. In an open letter in *The Oklahoma Veterinarian* that same year, Helen, in explaining why she paid her dues to the association said, "I have been proud of the fact that I am a Veterinarian and proud of having been the wife of a Veterinarian and wished to contribute my small share!"

After Patrick left for college, Helen sold the house she had shared with her family and moved to a smaller home. She stayed in Oklahoma for a few years, later moving back to Omaha when her health deteriorated.

After a lengthy battle with cancer, Helen passed away March 18, 1990.

Helen was a devoted mother, wife and grandmother.

Dr. Helen "Richt" Irwin, the girl from Sarpy County, will be remembered for her kind and loving ways. She was a woman with great determination who was not afraid to challenge new ground.

A child of the Depression, she lived for each new day, always willing to share her great knowledge of the profession when some young girl would ask. Helen was a wonderful person who has left an indelible mark on the face of women in veterinary medicine. She was a woman of few words according to her son Tom, but one saying she had that she might have left us with is, "It's a great life if you don't weaken."

The Dr. Helen Irwin Scholarship in Veterinary Medicine was established in 1990 to honor the historical significance of her being the first female graduate in veterinary medicine at Kansas State College.

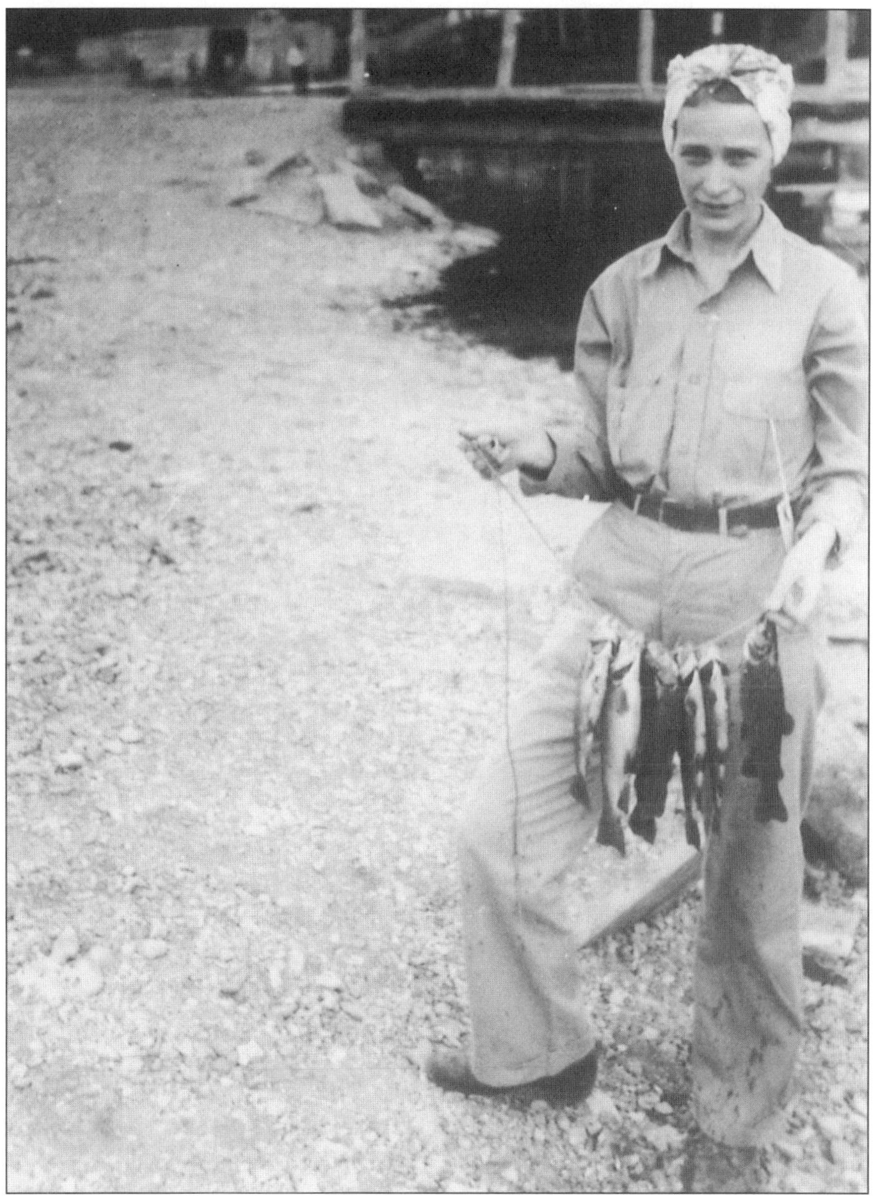

Helen fishing on one of the family's camping trips

Helen Richt
Chronology

1910: 9 October, born in Omaha, Nebraska.

1928: Graduated from South Omaha High School, Omaha, Nebraska.
10 September, *First woman* to be admitted to the professional curriculum. Kansas State College, Division of Veterinary Medicine.

1929: February, featured in the Jen-Sal Journal.
(Photograph used on front cover of this book.)

1932: Awarded the Franklin Prize in Pathology (O. M. Franklin donor, KSC 1912.)
2 June, Graduated from the professional curriculum, Kansas State College, Division of Veterinary Medicine.

1933: W. F. Irwin graduated D.V.M, from Division of Veterinary Medicine, Kansas State College. (Future husband of Helen Richt.)

1933-1934: Engaged as technician in the Pathology Laboratory, Kansas State College.

1934: 30 December, married to William F. Irwin.

1934-1935: Joined the faculty, Veterinary Division, Kansas State College.

1935: Purchased veterinary hospital in Tulsa, Oklahoma.

1937: First woman to hold an office in the A.V.M.A. Served as Secretary of the Section on Small Animals

24 April, son William born.

1940: 17 April, son Tom born.

1942: Opened the new City Veterinary Hospital, in South Tulsa, Oklahoma.

1945: 20 November, son Patrick born.

1955: Served as Secretary to the Oklahoma Veterinary Medical Association Auxiliary.

1959: 10 September, Helen's husband Dr. William F. Irwin, died in tragic accident in Alaska.

1960: Served as Treasurer to the Oklahoma Veterinary Medical Association.

1990: 18 March, Helen passed away in Omaha, Nebraska.

Division of Veterinary Medicine

Curriculum in Veterinary Medicine

1. Preveterinary Year[1]

(Thirty semester credits of approved college or university work, having the following distribution, are required.)

```
English..........................5 or 6 semester hours
General Inorganic Chemistry........5 to 10 semester hours
Zoölogy...........................5 semester hours
Military Science[2]................2 semester hours
Optional courses..................9 to 15 semester hours
                                  ———
    Total.........................30 or 32 semester hours
```

The optional courses should preferably be selected from a modern language (German or French), physics, and mathematics.

FRESHMAN

FIRST SEMESTER	SECOND SEMESTER
Anatomy I, Anat. 104..............*4(3-3)	Anatomy II, Anat. 110.............8(4-12)
Histology I, Path. 102.............4(2-6)	Histology II, Path. 106.............3(1-6)
Gen. Org. Chemistry, Chem. 122.....5(3-6)	Path. Bact. I, Bact. 111............4(2-6)
Medical Botany, Bot. 126..........2(1-3)	
Mil. Sci. (Vet.) I,[2] Mil. Tr. 121A...1(0-3)	Mil. Sci. (Vet.) II,[2] Mil. Tr. 122A...1(0-3)
Phys. Education M,[3] Phys. Ed. 103..R(0-2)	Phys. Education M,[3] Phys. Ed. 104..R(0-2)
Total......................... 16	Total......................... 16

SOPHOMORE

FIRST SEMESTER	SECOND SEMESTER
Anatomy III, Anat. 112.............4(1-9)	Pathology I, Path. 203.............5(3-6)
Comp. Physiology I, Anat. 222.....4(3-3)	Comp. Physiology II, Anat. 227.....4(3-3)
El. of An. Husb., An. Husb. 125.....3(2-4)	Farm Poultry Production, Poult. Husb.
	101 ....2(1-2, 1)
Path. Bact. II, Bact. 116...........4(2-6)	Feeding Live Stock, An. Husb. 172..3(3-0)
Dairy Cattle Judging, Dairy Husb.	Dairy Inspection II, Dairy Husb. 119, 2(1-3)
104 ....1(0-3)	
Mil. Sci. (Vet.) III,[4] Mil. Tr. 123A...1(0-3)	Mil. Sci. (Vet.) IV,[4] Mil. Tr. 124A...1(0-3)
Phys. Education M, Phys. Ed. 105...R(0-2)	Phys. Education M, Phys. Ed. 106..R(0-2)
Total...........................16 or 17	Total...........................16 or 17

JUNIOR

FIRST SEMESTER	SECOND SEMESTER
Surgery I, Surg. and Med. 102.......5(5-0)	Surgery II, Surg. and Med. 107......5(5-0)
Materia Medica, Surg. and Med. 158..4(3-3)	Dis. of Large Animals I, Surg. and
	Med. 175 ....5(5-0)
Pathology II, Path. 208.............4(3-3)	Pathology III, Path. 211............3(2-3)
Parasitology, Zoöl. 208 ....3(2-3)	Therapeutics, Surg. and Med. 163....3(3-0)
Clinics I, Surg. and Med. 138........2(0-6)	Clinics II, Surg. and Med. 141.......2(0-6)
Total......................... 18	Total......................... 18

SENIOR

FIRST SEMESTER	SECOND SEMESTER
Dis. of Large Animals II, Surg. and	Inf. Dis. of Large Animals, Surg. and
Med. 177 ....5(5-0)	Med. 181 ....5(5-0)
Dis. of Small Animals, Surg. and	Obstet. & Breeding Dis., Surg. and
Med. 186 ....2(2-0)	Med. 130 ....5(5-0)
Surgical Exercises, Surg. and Med.	Poultry Diseases, Bact. 217..........2(2-0)
112 ....1(0-3)	
Meat Hygiene, Path. 217............3(3-0)	Medical Economics & Law, Surg. and
Pathology IV, Path. 214............3(2-3)	Med. 190 ....2(2-0)
Clinics III, Surg. and Med. 144.....4(0-12)	Clinics IV, Surg. and Med. 147.....4(0-12)
Total......................... 18	Total......................... 18

```
Number of hours required in the preveterinary year............................. 32 or 30
Number of hours required in the freshman, sophomore, junior and senior years... 132 or 134

    Total number of hours required for graduation................................ 164
```

EXTRACURRICULAR ELECTIVES

FIRST SEMESTER	SECOND SEMESTER
	Special Histology, Path. 252........3(1-6)
Vaccine Manu. I, Path. 228........2(1-3)	Vaccine Manu. II, Path. 231........2(1-3)

FIRST OR SECOND SEMESTER

```
Pathological Technic and Diagnosis I, Path. 222..............2 to 5( - )
Pathological Technic and Diagnosis II, Path. 223.............2 to 5( - )
Research in Pathology, Path. 302............................1 to 10( - )
Special Anatomy, Anat. 202..................................2 to 4( - )
Applied Anatomy, Anat. 206....................................1(0-3)
Problems in Physiology, Anat. 215...........................3 to 5( - )
```

Veterinary Curriculum, 1932

Chapter 2

Louise Sklar
–1934 Division of Veterinary Medicine
Kansas State College

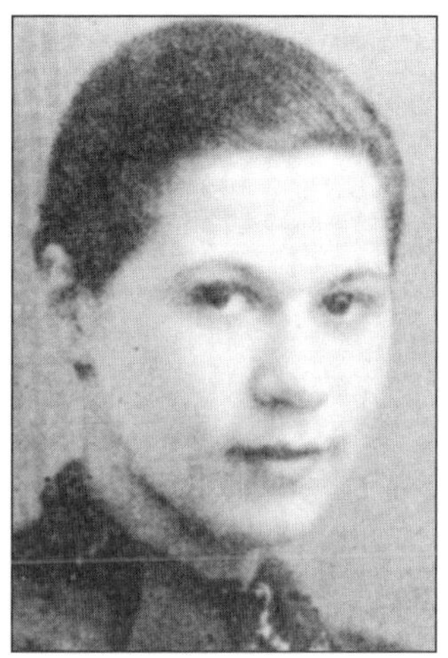

*L*ouise Sklar was the second daughter born to Russian immigrants Harry and Bessie Sklar. The Sklars and their daughters, Sadie, Louise and Ethel, and their son George, lived in Philadelphia, Pennsylvania. All the Sklar children were born in Philadelphia except for Ethel, who was born in Aurora, Nebraska, during a period of time when her parents were trying to establish a livelihood there. Louise attended the public schools and it was during her second year at Overbrook High School, in Philadelphia, that her parents were to move to Manhattan, Kansas.

Harry Sklar operated an auto-wrecking service, with his wife Bessie keeping the books. Bessie enjoyed being a home-maker to her family and later when war broke-out, she became a nurses-aide (scrub nurse). Bessie was proud to wear a uniform and be part of the war effort.

Even though the change from Philadelphia to Manhattan could have been a daunting one for a young Jewish teenager, Louise was not deterred. Louise's sister Ethel relates that maybe the welcome from a little boy in the neighborhood with a pet lamb was a sign that Louise was in the right place!

Louise loved animals and probably disappointed her parents as they were hoping that one day she would become a medical doctor. Louise was hooked on animals and was determined that she was going to become a veterinarian.

The exceptionally bright, young Louise had no problems in finishing her last two years of schooling at Manhattan High School. Having skipped a couple of years in elementary school back in Philadelphia, Louise was admitted to The Division of Veterinary Medicine, at Kansas State College, a few days before her fifteenth birthday. *(At this time, completion of college prerequisites prior to being admitted to veterinary school were not required).*

Veterinary school was good to Louise; she enjoyed the classes and her fellow class members. Being popular and having a great personality were attributes that helped tremendously in a class with thirty-nine men!

Manhattan was a good place to live and The Sklars enjoyed their time in the community. The population of Manhattan being approximately twenty-thousand, with the college enrolling approximately four thousand students, made for a community that appealed to the intelligentsia.

The Sklars home, 210 South 17th Street, was a house full of laughter and music, and was one that enjoyed company. It was also a great vantage point for the many impressive parades that would pass by from Fort Riley, which was a cavalry post in those days.

Louise's sister Ethel remembers her sister fondly, "Louise was warm, friendly, funny and although she was very smart, she wasn't 'nerdy.' She was a good sister and mentor to me." Louise started college when she was so young, that even she had said afterwards that she was not as mature socially as she was academically. However, she soon learned to keep up with her classmates and current fads in style, music, dancing, bridge etc. Being two years younger, it was a sad time for Ethel when Louise graduated and engaged in her new profession!

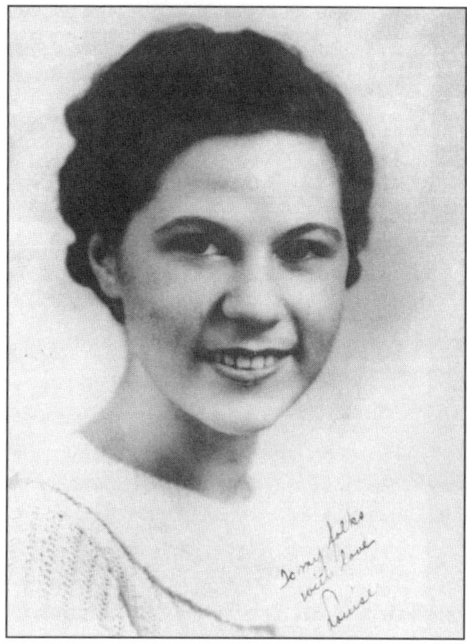

Dr. Louise Sklar

It was on May 31, 1934 that the eighteen year old Louise graduated with her veterinary degree, alongside thirty-nine male class members. Harry and Bessie Sklar were proud of their daughter, Louise' accomplishments. Their excitement continued as Sadie graduated as an Architect, from Kansas State, the same year. But in a few months, what should have been an exciting time in the lives of the Sklar family was marred by a tragic accident resulting in the untimely death of Sadie. Louise, Sadie and two friends had been en-route to a after-graduation party in Lincoln, Nebraska, when the car they were riding in blew a tire, causing the car to go out of control. Sadie laid in a coma for four days, before passing away August 18, 1934. Louise and their friends survived the accident with minor injuries.

Life would never be the same in the Sklar house-hold. The laughter changed into tears and many years passed before the family could be consoled.

Nevertheless, the young Louise moved on with her new profession. For the 1934-1935 school year she became an assistant to Dean Dykstra, Division of Veterinary Medicine, Kansas State College, teaching classes in anatomy for one semester.

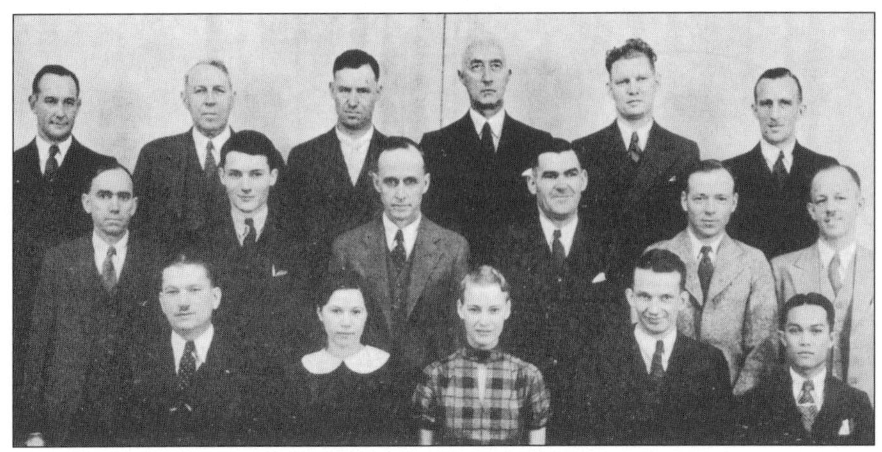

Dr. Louise Sklar with faculty, in 1934 -1935

The August, 1934 edition of *"Veterinary Medicine"* featured an article that Louise wrote about keeping a professional diary. She had learned in veterinary college that keeping good records were an important part of becoming a veterinarian. The article outlined what complete case records should include: Printed letterhead of the establishment, serial number and date, symptoms, diagnosis or tentative diagnosis, prognosis, all of which should be exact and in detail, so as to prevent misunderstandings at a later date. The article went on to mention that such records may serve other purposes than those for which they were intended! For instance; it *happened that a man accused of bank robbery in Denver testified that on the day on which the crime was committed, he was in Manhattan and had presented a German shepherd dog for treatment at the veterinary clinic of the Kansas State College. Complete case records at the clinic enabled the authorities to verify the alibi and he was freed of suspicion!*

The article was a staunch picture of how Louise conducted herself as a veterinarian, a professional in the true sense!

In the summer 1935, Louise resigned her position at Kansas State College, and moved to Fort Worth, Texas, where she assumed a temporary position with the United States Bureau of Animal Industry. She took immediate charge of the Bang's Abortion Disease Laboratory.

Dr. Louise Sklar was cited as America's youngest woman veterinarian in the "Fort Worth Star-Telegram," dated July 17, 1935! The article mentioned that Louise had become a veterinary student as a sort of pre-medicine work, but was so fascinated by it that she had to finish it. She stated: "It's interesting and I like it."

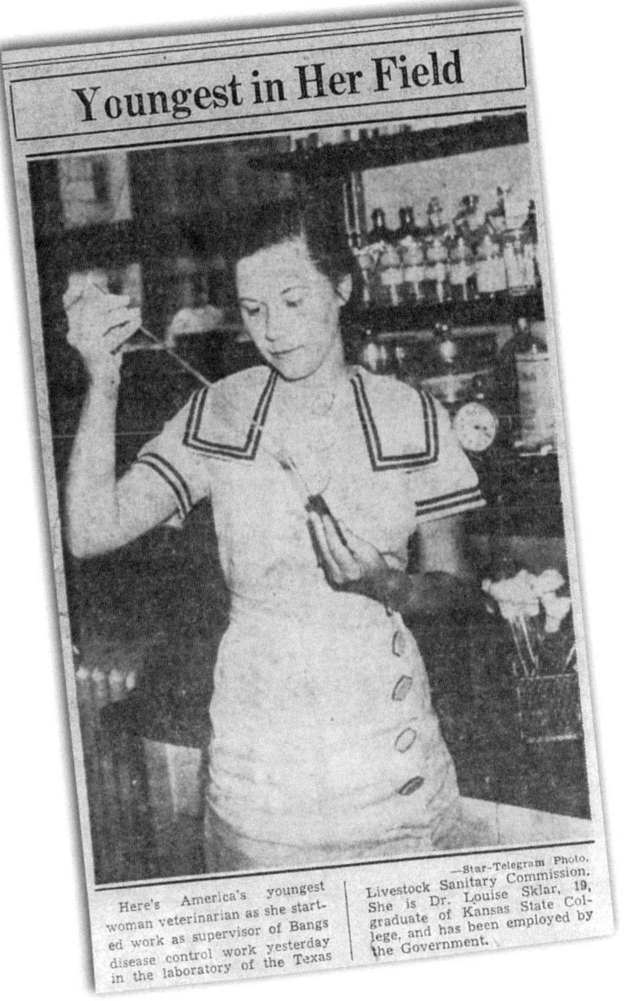

Here's America's youngest woman veterinarian as she started work as supervisor of Bangs disease control work yesterday in the laboratory of the Texas Livestock Sanitary Commission. She is Dr. Louise Sklar, 19, graduate of Kansas State College, and has been employed by the Government.

—Star-Telegram Photo.

Dr. Louise Sklar, *Youngest in Her Field*, newspaper clipping.

Her interest for veterinary medicine was *'heightened'* one year later in 1936, when she returned to Manhattan, Kansas, to work on her Masters Degree. The title of her Master's thesis was <u>*Absorption of Glucose from the Stomach of the Dog*</u>. She received her Master's degree 30 July, 1937.

Late in 1937 she began a two-year course of study to earn a Graduate Fellow from the University of Maryland in Research and General Laboratory Procedures. Louise was proud to receive the honor from Sigma Alpha Omega (*Bacteriology Honory Society*), upon her graduation from the University of Maryland. It was during her time at the University of Maryland where she met and eventually married Dr. Melvin Rabstein.

The next few years were spent working and starting a family. Melvin and Louise were blessed on December 2, 1940, with the arrival of their firstborn, a baby girl, Jeanne. A second baby girl, Susan, would arrive 12 October, 1943, born in Washington, DC.

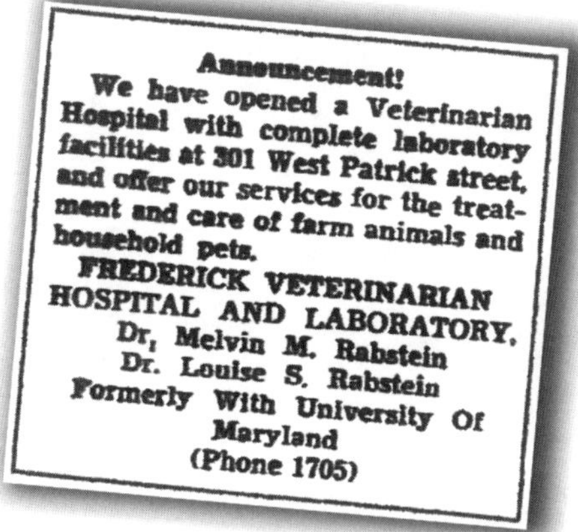

Announcement!
We have opened a Veterinarian Hospital with complete laboratory facilities at 301 West Patrick street, and offer our services for the treatment and care of farm animals and household pets.
FREDERICK VETERINARIAN HOSPITAL AND LABORATORY.
Dr. Melvin M. Rabstein
Dr. Louise S. Rabstein
Formerly With University Of Maryland
(Phone 1705)

Advertisement in the Frederick News, 1944

In 1944, Louise started a practice with her husband Dr. Melvin Rabstein, a 1937 graduate of the University of Pennsylvania School of Veterinary Medicine. The couple shared the responsibilities of their new practice in Frederick, Maryland, Louise working on small animals and Melvin on the large animals. It was not unusual to see Louise de-scenting skunks or working on monkeys from a local carnival. She enjoyed whatever was put in front of her. Evenings were spent with their children, sometimes sharing it with any necessary surgeries! A third 'assistant', baby girl Linda, was born October 4, 1946.

Louise had achieved entering a profession that was, at the time, considered to be a man's profession: She had overcome the obstacles and was accomplished in all that she undertook. Louise was proud of this and chose to pass on her wealth of knowledge; in 1951 she became a charter member of the Soroptomist International. *(Soroptimist is an international volunteer service organization for business and professional women who work to improve the lives of women and girls, in local communities and throughout the world.)* She served as Vice President, and in due course, was elected in 1954 as director. Louise championed such causes as: The Polio campaign, United Nations, Home for the Aged, and many more.

Louise took advantage of any situation where she could voice her opinion about women in veterinary medicine. In one meeting for the Soroptomist club in November, 1953, she delivered a talk; her topic being, "The Place of Women in Veterinary Medicine."

"The prevention of disease is more important than the cure," Dr. Rabstein told her audience. She mentioned that, although it is a difficult and limited field, she found it very rewarding. She listed disease study, mode of transmission, education of public as the matter in which veterinarians can most effectively protect their cause. She also discussed in detail means of controlling such diseases as undulant fever and tuberculosis, often transmitted from animal to human. Dr. Rabstein was proud to mention that she was one of two women veterinarians in the state of Maryland, and that there were only 200 women graduates of veterinary medicine in the United States and Canada at this time.

Louise and her husband sold their practice in the mid - 1960's. For awhile, Louise stayed at home enjoying knitting, dancing, cooking and taking art classes, until she was offered a job in research.

Her work as a researcher for Microbiological Associates, in Bethesda, Maryland, earned Louise wide recognition as a scientist. In a few short years, from approximately 1968–1973, she co–authored more than a dozen papers on her work on cancer. Sadly, a paper entitled *Multiple Spontaneous Tumors in BALB/cf/Cd Mice*, was the last paper she wrote.

During a routine physical, indications of lung cancer were found and surgery performed. It was after a brave battle that Louise's life ended 10 August, 1973. She was 57 years old.

Dr. Louise (Sklar) Rabstein was not to be forgotten. Her final paper was presented posthumously, at the Fifth Perugia Quadrennial International Conference on Cancer, in Italy, the following year 1974.

Her name and works were cited in "American Men and Women of Science," Twelfth edition, "Who's Who of American Women," Eighth edition, and "Who's Who, 1973."

Louise will be remembered as probably being the youngest female to enter veterinary school at Kansas State College, but first and foremost as a leader in physical, biological, and related sciences, of which she would have been proud!

THE LADY IS A VETERINARIAN

Louise Sklar
Chronology

1915: 23 September, Louise Sklar was born to Russian immigrants Harry and Bessie Sklar, Philadelphia, Pennsylvania. Louise had one older sister Sadie, one younger sister Ethel, and baby brother George. Attended public schools, including Overbrook High School, Philadelphia, Pennsylvania.

1928: Summer, moved with family to Manhattan, Kansas. 10, September, entered Manhattan High School.

1930: 22 May, graduated high school at 14 years of age. 9, September, admitted to Professional Curriculum, Division of Veterinary Medicine, Kansas State College. Member of the Student Chapter American Veterinary medical Association.

1934: 31 May, graduated with D.V.M. along-side thirty-nine men, Kansas State College. 8 August, sister Sadie Sklar killed in auto accident near Beatrice, Nebraska.

1934-1935: Taught for one semester as assistant to Dean Dykstra, Division of Veterinary Medicine, Kansas State College.

1935: In charge of Bang's Laboratory, Fort Worth, Texas.

1936-1937: Graduate Work, Kansas State College. 30 July, graduated with M.S. degree in Physiology, Kansas State College.

1937-
1939 : Graduated fellow at the University of Maryland - Research and General Lab. Procedures (College Park., Maryland). Met and married Dr. Melvin Rabstein.

1940 : 2 December, baby daughter Jeanne, their first-born, Hyattsville, Maryland.

1943 : 12 October, a second baby girl Susan, born in Washington, D.C.

1944 : Engaged in practice with husband Dr. Melvin Rabstein, Frederick, Maryland.

1946 : 4 October, baby girl Linda born.

1959 : 16 January, Bessie Sklar passed away.
26 February, Harry Sklar passed away.

1966 : Circa: sold veterniary practice, Frederick, Maryland.

1968 : Started work as scientist for Microbiological Associates, Bethesda, Maryland.

1973 : Died 10 August, NIH Hospital, Bethesda, Maryland. Place of Interment: Frederick, Maryland, age 57. Survived by her widow, three daughters, one brother, one sister, and three grandchildren.

Chapter 3

Hautesse "Tess" Etoile Rondeau
–1944 School of Veterinary Medicine
Kansas State College

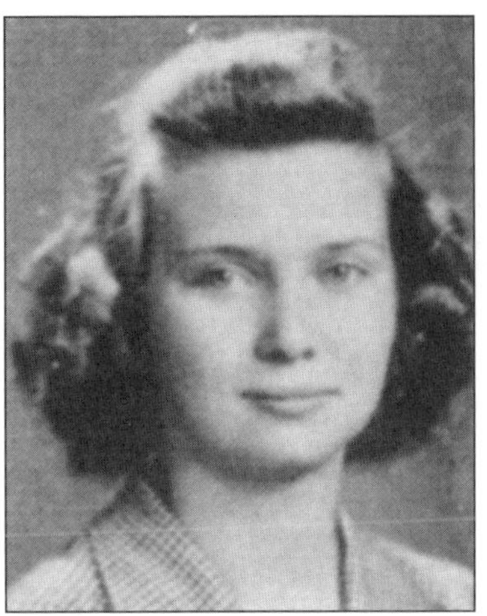

*H*autesse Etoile Rondeau was born on the Twentieth of February, 1921, in Shreveport, Louisiana. She was the eldest of three children born to Henri and Beatrice Rondeau. Hautesse would spend her elementary years growing up in Shreveport with her sister Dolores and younger brother Henri.

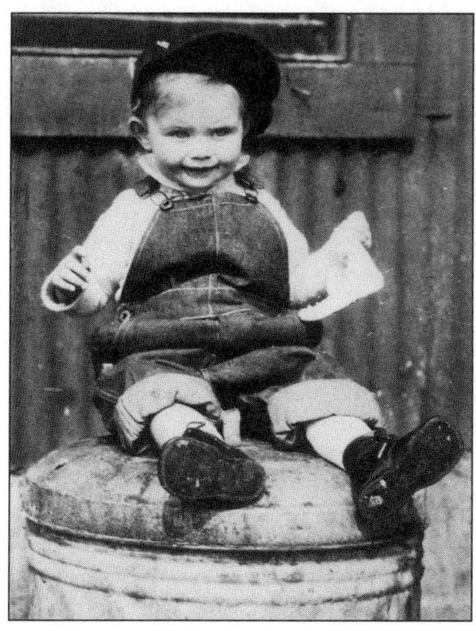

Tess at home in Shreveport, circa 1922

Hautesse's parents had met in August of 1915 in Eagle Pass, Texas. Her father, a 'land man,' was into oil exploration throughout Kansas, Texas, Oklahoma and Louisiana. Henri was of French - Canadian heritage, but did not speak French. Beatrice (Spraugh) Rondeau, a beautiful well - dressed young woman, was from Great Bend, Kansas. The many photographs in the cherished scrapbook that Hautesse's grandmother started for her show a well dressed and cultured family.

The love Hautesse had for animals was apparent during her childhood. She was often seen riding the family's pet Borzoi, a Russian Wolfhound. Her father encouraged her love for animals and bought Hautesse a goat and cart when she was three years old. A Boston terrier and a Labrador were also fondly remembered as family pets.

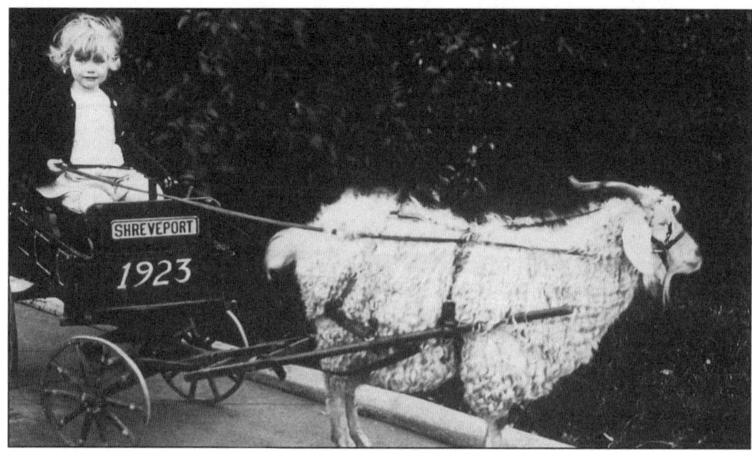

Tess in her goat cart, circa 1923

One person who gave much love and encouragement to Hautesse was 'Grandpa Spraugh,' her mother's father. C. D. Spraugh owned a grocery store on Main Street in Great Bend, Kansas. Grandpa Spraugh wrote to Hautesse while she was in Shreveport, always encouraging her to do well in school.

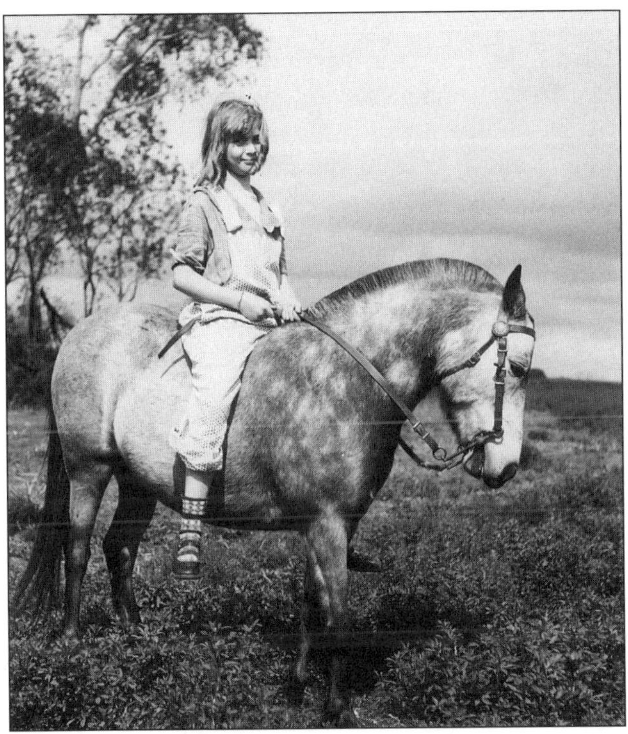

Tess riding horse in Great Bend, Kansas

Another relative, Hautesse's uncle "Brit Spraugh," a man of great character, also had great support for Hautesse. His love for the many animals that he collected for his zoo at Great Bend, Kansas, would also be an inspiration to Hautesse.

In 1930 Beatrice Rondeau moved with her three children to Great Bend, Kansas. They lived with her parents at the grocery store on Main Street. Hautesse enjoyed this time and remembers helping to stock the shelves at the store for her grandfather.

"Tess," as she is better known to her friends, excelled in her school-work, receiving many awards of honor for her good work. She graduated from Great Bend High School in 1939. Having worked hard and receiving excellent grades she was admitted to the Pre-veterinary Curriculum in September 1939 and the Professional Curriculum in 1940 at Kansas State College, School of Veterinary Medicine.

Tess spent her time in veterinary school working hard at her studies and working part-time at a local cafeteria where she would work early in the morning as a cashier and wash pots and pans late at night. Tess remembers her time in veterinary school as a pleasant challenge. She shared her days in the classroom with twenty-seven men and one other woman, Louise Scherger.

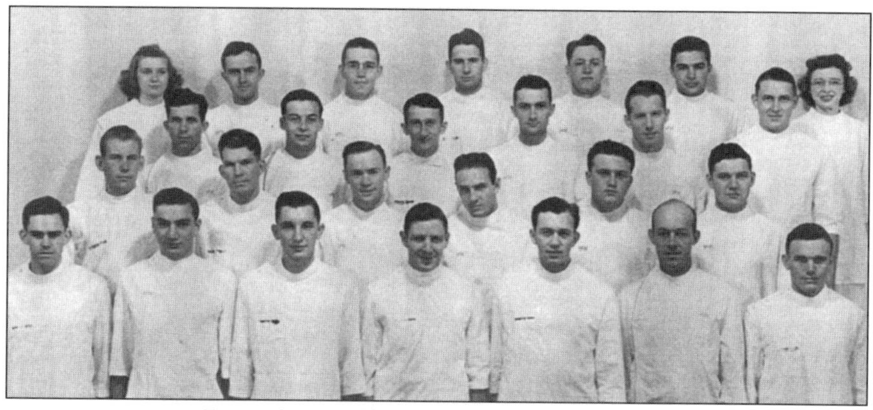

Tess and some of her classmates, her senior year

Tess spent any spare time she had studying, as she knew that to attain the dream she had as a young child she would have to work hard. Whilst in veterinary school she belonged to the Student Chapter of the AVMA and was an active member of the American Rabbit Breeders Association.

During the time Tess was in veterinary school many changes took place. In 1942 the "accelerated" program was introduced. This meant the students had year round instruction enabling their training to be completed in three years, rather than four. This also meant that for certain years there would be two graduating classes.

While in veterinary school, Tess was randomly selected and assigned to the M.A.C Reserve. The Medical Administrative Corps was established in June, 1920. *(The concept of the M.A.C. was to have a cadre of ancillary medical professionals to free doctors for their professional practices.)* Even though Tess was not called to duty, it was an honor to be included in a Corps that's history can be traced as early as the American War of Independence.

Tess remembers the walk from her home on North Fourteenth Street in Manhattan to the veterinary school as a time of relaxation. Enjoying the scenic campus made her feel good about her long days in school. She remembered when, on one cold day walking to school, a young family pulled up in their car to offer her a ride, which she willingly accepted. She was asked by one of the young ladies in the car where she was going, when she replied 'to my classes at the veterinary school,' the young lady told Tess that she thought that being in veterinary school was not the place for ladies! Tess never could understand why the young lady thought that way.

Tess enjoyed her classes and even when she was in the midst of a classroom dispute because of her gender, she stayed strong. "Anatomy classes were always a problem," Tess has told me. It was Dr. R. H. Burt head of the Anatomy and Physiology Dept, who defended Tess, by explaining that she had every right to be in the classroom with the men. Apparently, one of Tess's classmates had not scored well on a test and he blamed Tess because he said that it was hard for the men to express certain anatomical parts in front of a lady! This was something that Tess had to deal with on a daily basis. The situation in the classroom became a little better once Dean Ralph Dykstra reiterated Dr. Burt's point of view!

For the most part, the men accepted Tess and her fellow lady class-mate well. The late Dr. Wesley Wertz wrote to tell me, "He thought both Tess and Louise were both congenial classmates." He was sure that life was not easy going to school with the boys. They were good sports and good students. He remembered Tess as being quite outgoing and in large animal clinics; that she was kept busy in swine obstetrics because of her small hands!

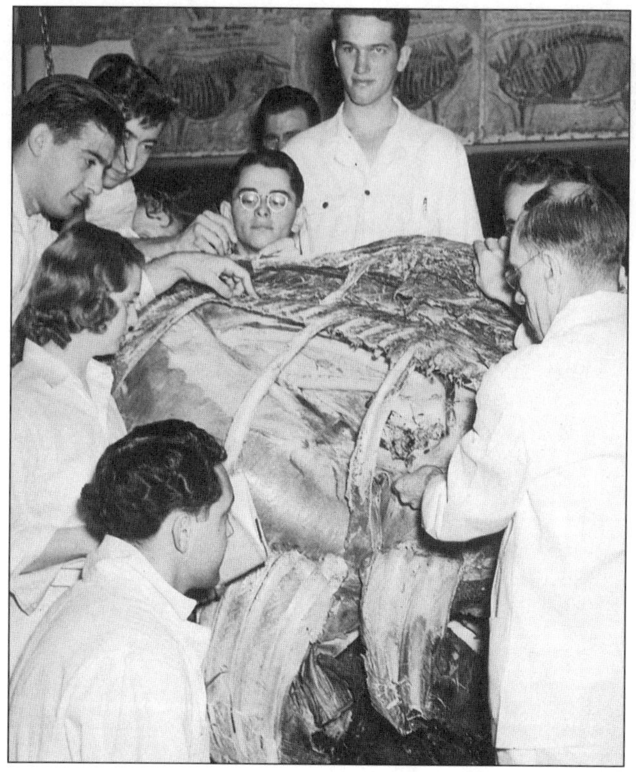

Tess with the men in Anatomy Class

There was no way that anyone could have thought that the hard working, five foot-one inch, blue-eyed and attractive female with the brown hair would not to achieve her dream!

It was on the Sixteenth Day of September, 1944 that Tess's dream came to fruition. On this day alongside twenty seven men and one other woman, the degree in veterinary medicine was conferred to Tess.

Tess spent her first few months out of school working for Dr. A. V. Young in Shreveport, Louisiana. Her career was put on hold after she contracted Tuberculosis. She spent two years recovering in sanitariums in Kansas and Louisiana. This was a blow to the vivacious young woman who had worked so hard in school to fulfill her dream, and was now sick!

It was 1946 before she was well enough to return to veterinary practice. Tess returned to her home in Great Bend, Kansas to work for Dr. Jay Reynolds, (KSU 1942).

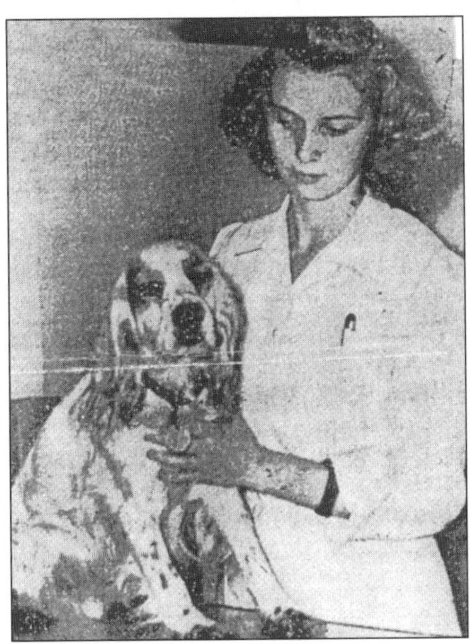

Dr. Hautesse Rondeau in practice, Great Bend, Kansas

Tess's dream of veterinary practice was becoming jaded. She was not as well accepted as she would have liked. She knew she was not always liked in veterinary school because of her gender, but to be a professional and disliked was beginning to ware on her!

Tess enjoyed her patients who were not swayed by her gender, but some of their owner's were concerned. It was not proper for a lady to be up to her armpits in manure, or working on sows laying face-down in the barn! Tess returned to her Alma Mater to visit with her friends in hope that they would boost her feelings of dismay!

It was in 1949, after two years working with Dr. Reynolds, that Tess wanted to return to Louisiana. She was an associate to the late Dr. L. P. Caraway (KSU 1925), and his son Dr. Hugh L. Caraway (KSU 1943) at the Caraway Veterinary Hospital, Shreveport, LA.

Tess enjoyed being back home in Shreveport with familiar faces, but alas, once again not all were receptive to a lady veterinarian. It became very clear to Tess that the farmers would never tolerate a woman treating their animals. Considering that the greater percentage of veterinary work at this time was on livestock left Tess feeling very unhappy. She occasionally saw small animals in the hospital, but it was a time when nobody thought you should pay to have your pet worked on!

Sadly, Tess decided to change her profession. She returned to school to become a Medical Lab Technician at the Confederate Memorial Medical Center which later became LSU Medical Center Hospital. Tess worked under Dr. W. R. Mathews (Pathologist), at Confederate, from 1956 until her retirement in 1979. She enjoyed this work and even though she was only one woman in the lab at first, she was proud of her new profession. Her time at Kansas State College, would never be forgotten, she would always be proud to have graduated a D.V.M.!

Tess established her home, a beautiful log house in Bossier City, Louisiana where she has enjoyed her family, friends and her many animals. Even though she missed being a practicing veterinarian she had many animals of her own to take care of. She adopted burros from the Grand Canyon and also had a small herd of Charolais cows. The cow herd's health was entrusted to her veterinarian Dr. Ronnie L. Powers (Auburn 1970).

Dr. Power's was joined in marriage and his practice by Dr. Sue Bradley in 1993. Dr. Bradley became a good friend of Tess's. She remembers Tess coming to the clinic with one of her poodles. Tess had an appointment with Dr. Power's, who like most large animal veterinarians was late! Dr. Bradley

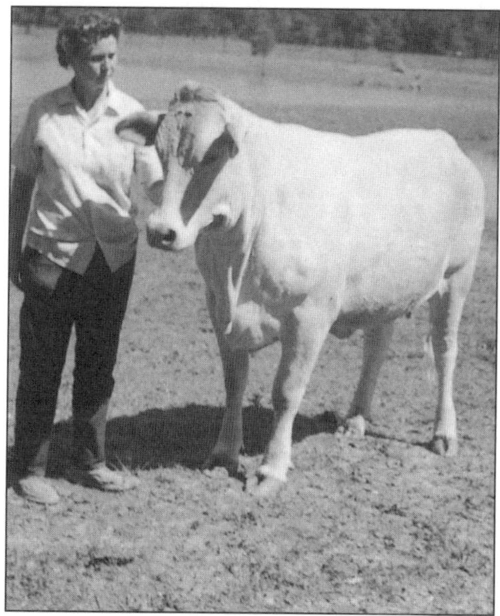

Tess with one of her cows, circa 1965

who had been showing Tess around the clinic offered to look at the little dog Scarlet, but Tess declined and said she'd wait for Dr. Powers, he was used to looking at Scarlet. Dr. Bradley carried on showing Tess the blood machines, heartworm tests, all the new things Tess had never seen whilst in practice. Finally Tess said, "Well I guess it'd be good for you to give Scarlet her vaccinations, I've never known a man who could stay on schedule!"

When Tess was about 65 years old, still strong and able, she was able to become a *practicing veterinarian* once again. After finding her cows down on the ground seizuring, she called for Dr. Powers' help. On his arrival, Tess assisted treating the cows as Dr. Powers prescribed. It was sad to lose seven or eight of her cows, but gratifying to save thirty that were treated. Tess found out that the pecan tree's surrounding her property had been sprayed with Thiodan, and she was not told to move her cattle. Tess was compensated for her loss and all was well. Dr. Powers always remembered his assistant Tess, "running from cow to cow crying as she tried to save them."

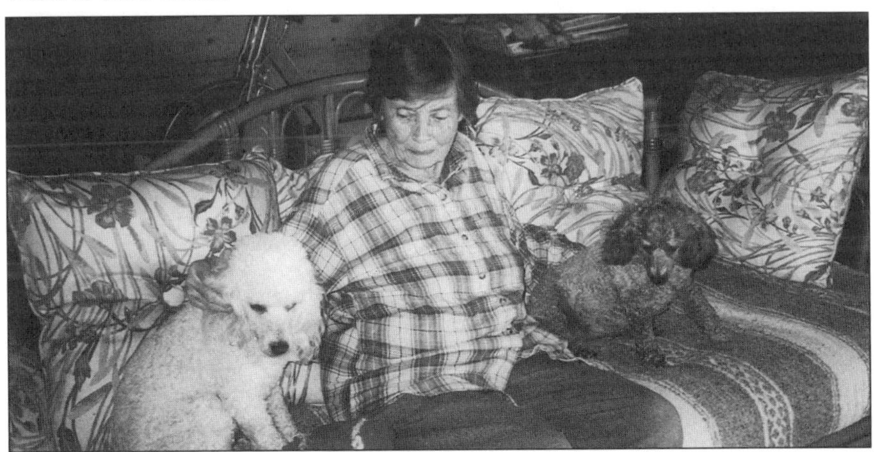

Tess with Louie and Scarlet, at home in Bossier City, Louisiana

As she sit's with her two best friend's, her poodles, Louie and Scarlet, there will never be a time that she will forget how proud she is to be a veterinarian, if only for awhile!!

THE LADY IS A VETERINARIAN

Hautesse Etoile Rondeau
Chronology

1921 : February 20, Hautesse Etoile Rondeau was born in Shreveport, Louisiana, to Ebert and Beatrice (Spraugh) Rondeau.

1939 : Graduated from Great Bend High School, Great Bend, Kansas. September, admitted to Pre - veterinary curriculum at Kansas State College.

1940 : Admitted to the Professional Curriculum at Kansas State College, School of Veterinary Medicine.

1942 : June 24, assigned to the M. A. C Reserve.

1944 : September 16, 1944 Dr. Hautesse Rondeau graduates D.V.M. from Kansas State College, School of Veterinary Medicine.

Dr. Rondeau would be associated in practice with Dr. A. V. Young, Shreveport, LA.

*1944-
1946* : Contracted TB, recuperated in sanitariums in Kansas and Louisiana.

*1946-
1948* : Practiced with Dr. Jay Reynolds at the Reynolds Veterinary Hospital in Great Bend, Kansas.

1947 : Father passed away in Monroe, Louisinana.

1949 : Practiced with Dr. L. P Caraway, (Veterinary Division KSU 1925) and his son Dr. Hugh L. Caraway (KSCSVM July 1943) in Shreveport, Louisiana.

1956 : Started work as Medical Lab Technician, at the Confederate Memorial Medical Center, (which would later become LSU Medical Center Hospital).

1967 : Dr. Rondeau's Mother, Beatrice Rondeau passed away.

1979 : Retired from LSU Medical Center.

1979-Present : Resides in Bossier City, Louisiana.

Chapter 4

Louise Ann Scherger
–1944 School of Veterinary Medicine
Kansas State College

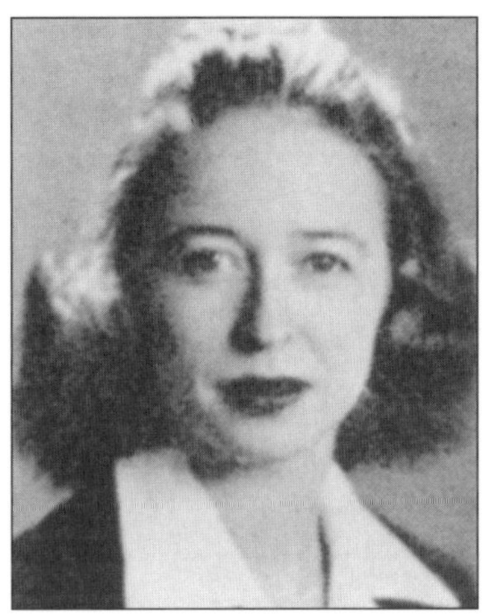

$\mathcal{L}$ouise Ann Scherger, the only child of Herman Bernard Scherger and Rosa May "Kunzel" Scherger, was born on November 11, 1921, in Wichita, Kansas.

Growing up for young Louise was a lonely time. Her mother worked as a seamstress in Wichita, and her father worked on oil exploration.

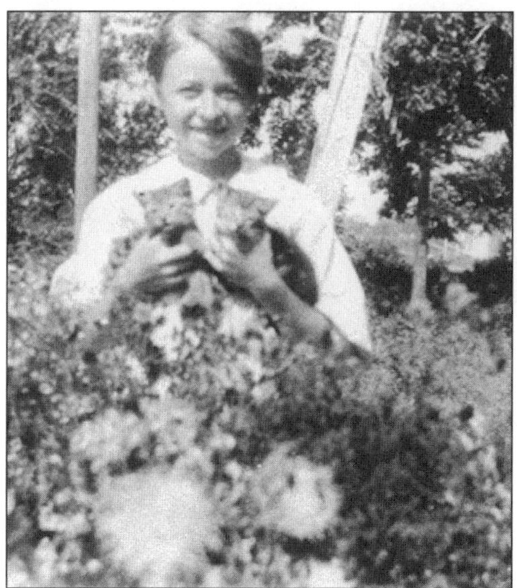

Louise with Umber and Ella

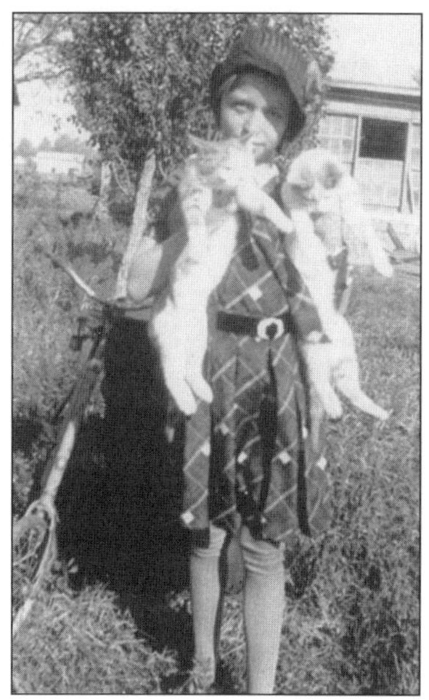

Louise with friends on
her tenth birthday

Louise and her family lived on a farm in Valley Center, Kansas. Her father had a reputation for 'brawling,' which meant that friends were not allowed to play with Louise!

Louise, as a teenager, sadly had to witness her father take his life. It was hard for her to be remorseful after all the years of anguish her father had put both her and her mother through.

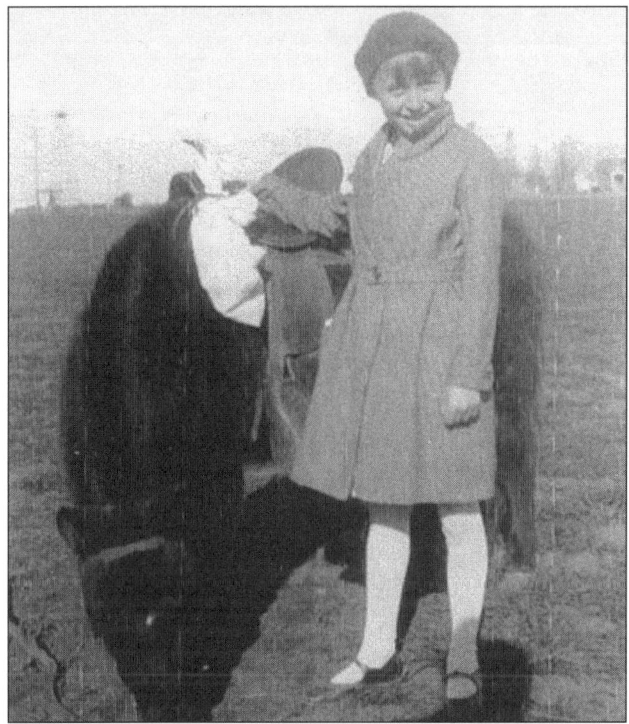

Louise with pony Beandy, circa 1933

Louise, being a smart and bright young woman, was eager to make good in her life. She worked hard in school to attain good grades. She attended Cathedral High School in Wichita, and Mount St. Scholastica, in Atchinson, Kansas.

Following her graduation from high school she entered the University of Wichita.

Louise enjoyed the sciences and animals so she decided to apply to veterinary school at Kansas State College. She was happy to be accepted, and entered into the professional curriculum in September of 1941.

The petite, red-blonde Louise stayed busy, enjoying most of her classmates. The classmates she did not like she avoided.

Louise was in one of the classes that, during wartime, that permitted her to graduate after three years, providing she achieved all required classes.

Louise enjoyed the one other female in her class, Hautesse Rondeau. They were of great encouragement to each other when the going was tough. Realizing they were pursuing a 'male dominated' profession, they had to work harder to prove their place in the class. They were not easily discouraged, they were determined young women!

When Louise was not studying in vet school, she devoted her time to community efforts. It seemed that from the long list of activities she pursued, maybe she was making up for lost time with friends! Louise was a member of the Newman Catholic Club, joining with others of her faith to socialize, educate and enjoy fellowship together.

She was active in the Y.M.C.A., participating in many campus projects, including freshman fellowship, leadership councils and interest groups.

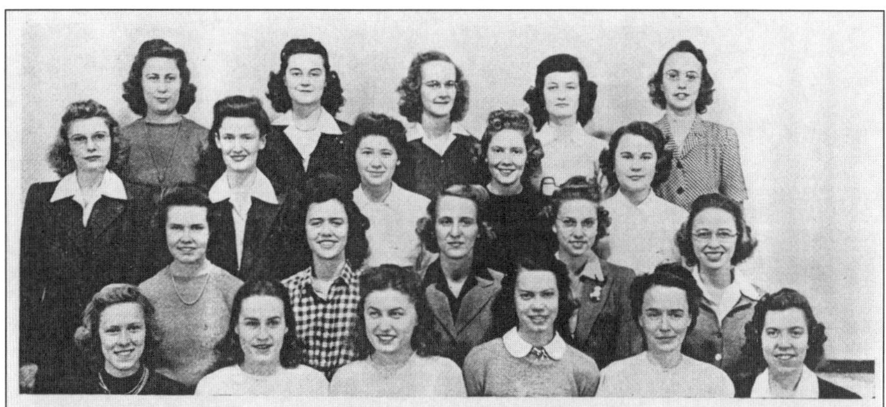

Y.W.C.A. CABINET—*Back row*: Betty J. Babb, Marjorie F. Correll, Mary F. Isely, Roberta M. Townley, Virginia L. Slothower. *Third row*: Ruth Catherine King, Ethelinda E. Parrish, Edith H. Willis, Faye Jean Gleason, Margaret McNamee. *Second row*: Lois E. Johnson, O. Jean Kays, Betty Brass, Alice Roelfs, Louise Scherger. *Front row*: Margaret E. Giles, Judy W. Doryland, Victoria Majors, Betty L. Payne, Dorothy M. Downey, Maxine Smith.

Louise was proud to be initiated into Alpha Delta Pi, a sisterhood that is committed to high academic standards, values, ethics and social responsibility.

Louise was marshal of Prix, an honor society for junior women that stressed scholarship and leadership.

Maybe it was her ancestors' 'bohemian' influence that pushed her to excel, regardless, Louise was not afraid to achieve.

Wesley Wertz, a classmate in the same group as Louise and Hautesse, remembers that Louise was a good sport and good student. He noted that life was not easy, for the 'ladies' to be in a class with some forty-eight men! Wesley felt honored to be in a class with the women!

Louise, alongside one woman and twenty-seven men, accepted her D.V. M. on September 16, 1944.

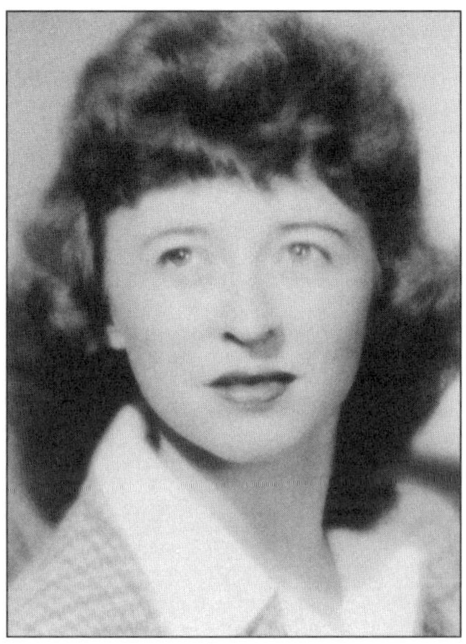

Dr. Louise Scherger, circa 1945

Dr. Louise Scherger's professional career started in Minneapolis, Minnesota, as an associate veterinarian at Morgan Hospital. After a year she moved to Omaha, Nebraska, to work as assistant veterinarian for the Corn States Serum Co.

Once again in 1946, Louise wanting to further her career, returned to school at the University of Wisconsin. She worked as a pathology instructor in the veterinary science department while working and researching for her Masters degree of which she received in 1947.

It was at the University of Wisconsin that she met and married Charles Lombard. Charles, like Louise, was a PhD student who eventually became a Professor of French.

Charles and Louise were blessed September 21, 1949 with their first-born, a baby girl Rhian.

Dr. Louise "Scherger" Lombard earned her PhD in Medical Pathology April 1, 1950. Louise enjoyed the challenges of her profession and was always eager to share her knowledge with others. She was devoted, kind and compassionate.

Louise returned to teaching at the Woman's Medical College of Pennsylvania in 1950 through 1951. It was an honor for her to be associated with such a prestigious College. (The first women's medical college in the world, chartered and opened in 1851 as the Female Medical College of Pennsylvania).

In the January, 1950 issue of Journal of Morphology, a well written article, of which Louise was the senior author, "The Morphology of the Oviduct of Virgin Heifers in Relation to the Estrous Cycle," was published.

After one year at Woman's Medical College, Louise worked from 1951 through 1952 as a research associate in the Virology Department at the University of Pennsylvania.

Louise and husband Charles were kept busy the next few years with a son, Charles, born July 16, 1952. Two years later on October 14, 1954, their son Robert was born.

From 1952 through 1955, she was assistant professor in the Pathology Department, at the University of Pennsylvania.

Even though babies took precedence over work, Louise found time to write. She was junior author of a book entitled "Equine Infectious Anemia," published by the University of Pennsylvania Press.

Louise was proud to qualify for membership to the American College of Veterinary Pathologists in 1955. It was a great achievement for a woman at this time to receive Diplomate status.

Even though Louise had 'ploughed' through disparaging remarks from faculty in veterinary school about her being a woman in a 'man's field,' she felt compelled to pass on her talents to other women. Her opportunity came in 1956 through 1958 when she became

President of the American Women's Veterinary Medical Association, as it was then.

Louise in her 1958 Presidential message mentioned the importance of women uniting and using their talents to the best advantage. She went on to talk of opportunities for women within the veterinary profession. She encouraged women veterinarians to look at the field of animal laboratory research.

One of the highlights of Louise's career came in 1955 through 1957 when she became Biologist in the Pathology Laboratory, at the national Cancer Institute in Bethesda, Maryland. She was considered to be one of the country's foremost research scientists in the study of cancer.

Louise lost her mother Rosa May, to cancer in 1957. Louise, who had so much to thank her mother for, redoubled her efforts in cancer research.

Louise transferred to Argonne National Laboratories, near Chicago, Illinois, in 1957. It was here that she began studies on animals, such as snakes and gerbils that were known to tolerate high doses of radiation. Dr. Douglas Grahn, who was Senior Biologist at Argonne and colleague of Louise's, remembers her as being reliable, and excellent at her microscopic work.

Once again, on May 2, 1958, Louise and husband Charles were blessed with another son, James, completing their family.

For the next twenty or more years, Louise devoted her efforts to field of cancer research. At Argonne National Laboratory she worked as an associate scientist from 1957 through 1964, and later as a pathologist. She was honored many times in her career for her outstanding work.

She was extremely proud in 1963 to receive the Centennial Award for Distinguished Service from her veterinary school at Kansas State College.

Louise enjoyed her work to the point that she liked to challenge herself with new opportunities. In 1964 through 1966 she was the pathologist at the Chicago Zoological Park.

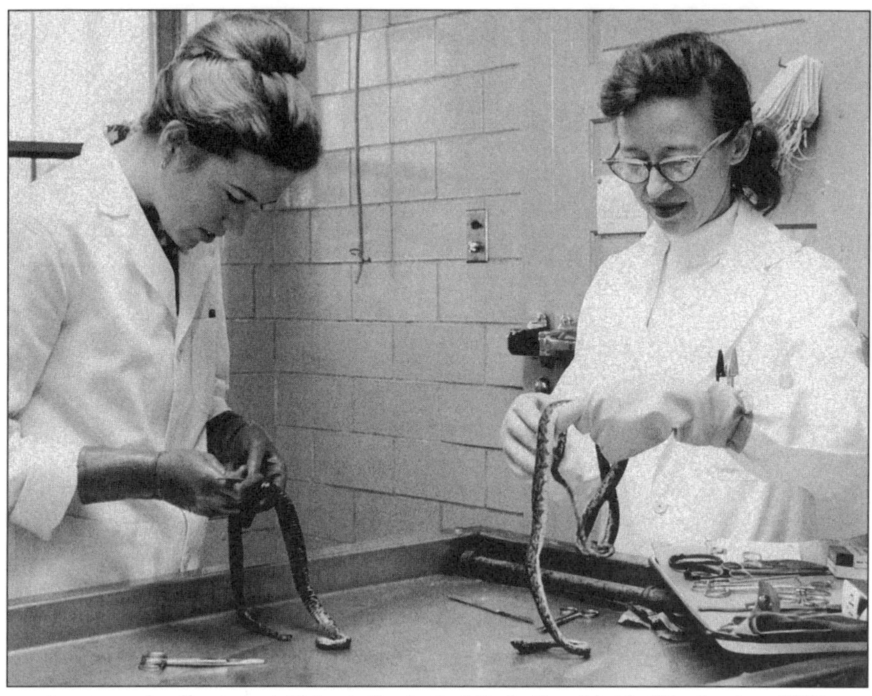

Louise and colleague, at Chicago Zoological Park, Brookfield, Illinois, circa 1965

Daughter Rhian remembers going to work with her Mom. She learned about dissecting animals, which in turn, she and her siblings demonstrated on their stuffed animals. Louise had taught them well!

Dr. Patricia "O'Connor" Halloran, America's first woman zoo veterinarian, remembered Louise as "one of the most delightful and accomplished people I have ever known."

Dr. O'Connor submitted many specimens, such as snakes, primates and big cats, for Louise to necropsy and evaluate.

Louise served on the faculties of Loyola Medical Center, in Illinois, from 1964 through 1969, and The University of Chicago from 1969 through 1972 respectively.

After two years working as head pathologist at Abbot Laboratories, in Illinois, continuing her research in cancer, Louise returned to Argonne National Laboratories.

In 1983 Louise was appointed to the Board of Scientific Counselors of the Division of Cancer Cause and Prevention of the National Cancer Institute.

It was a sad time for Louise and her family when in October of 1985, Charles Lombard passed away following a stroke.

Louise retired at age sixty-five, moving to California to be near family. In her spare time she enjoyed sewing, and working in her garden.

Louise sadly passed away August 2, 1987. She had left the most remarkable trail. Her contribution to veterinary science was outstanding, having authored and co-authored many scientific papers. She received an honorary degree from Harvard University. She traveled with a panel of experts to many international locations including Japan as part of the International Life Sciences Institute.

Louise would have been proud to know that she would be considered a modern day 'mentor.' She showed that it is possible to be a wife, mother and a hard working professional. She was as dedicated to her profession as any man. She truly paved a better path for all the women who followed!

THE LADY IS A VETERINARIAN

Louise Ann Scherger
Chronology

1921 : Born November 20, 1921, in Wichita, Kansas.

1938 : 16 May, Herman Scherger, Louise's father died

1941 : 8 Sepetember, admitted to the professional curriculum at KSCSVM. Member of Alpha Delta Pi.

1944 : 16 September, graduated D.V.M. KSCSVM.

1944-1945 : Associate Veterinarian, Morgan Hospital, Minneapolis, Minnesota.

1945-1946 : Assistant Veterinarian and Diagnostician, Corn States Serum Co., Omaha, Nebraska.

1946-1950 : Instructor in Veterinary Pathology, Veterinary Science Dept, University of Wisconsin, Madison

1948 : 21 June, married Charles M. Lombard

1949 : 21 September, firstborn baby girl Rhian

1950 : Earned PhD in Pathology, University of Wisconsin, Madison, Wisconsin.

1950-1951: Instructor, Department of Pathology, Woman's Medical College of Pennsylvania, Philadelphia.

1951-1952: Research Associate, Virology, University of Pennsylvania, Philadelphia

1952: 16 July, birth of son Charles

1954: 14 October, birth of son Robert

1955: Diplomate, American College of Veterinary Pathology

1955-1957: Biologist, Laboratory of Pathology, National Cancer Institute, Bethesda, Maryland

1957: Rosa May Scherger, Louise's mother, passed away.

1957-1964: 1 October, 1957, worked as Pathologist, at Argonne National Lab, until 31 August, 1964.

1958: 2 May, birth of son James
President of the Women's Veterinary Association

1959: Certificate in Radiation Biology, Argonne National Laboratory.

1960 : Postgraduate work in Electron Microscopy, Argonne National Laboratory.

1961 : Postgraduate work in Histochemistry, Northwestern University.

1963 : Received the Centennial Award for Distinguished Service, Kansas State College.

1964 : Diplomate, American College of Laboratory Medicine.

1964–1966 : Pathologist, Chicago Zoological Park, Brookfield, Illinois.

1964–1969 : Associate Professor, Department of Pathology, Loyola Medical Center, Maywood, Illinois.

1969–1972 : Associate Professor, Departments of Pathology and Pharmacology, The University of Chicago.

1972–1974 : Head, Pathology Section, Abbot Laboratories, Abbot Park, Illinois.

1974–1983 : 2 December, 1974, worked as Pathologist, at Argonne National Lab, until 30 November, 1983.

1984-1986: 16 January, 1984, worked as Pathologist/STA (Staff Temporary Appointment), until 2 August, 1987.

1985: 6 October, husband Charles passed away.

1987: 2 August, Dr. Louise "Scherger" Lombard, died in California.

1971/ 76/ 79/ 82/ 86/ 89/ 92/ 93/ 94/ 98/ 2003: Cited in American Men and Women of Science.

Chapter 5

Ordella Ida Geisler
–1947 Division of Veterinary Medicine
Kansas State College

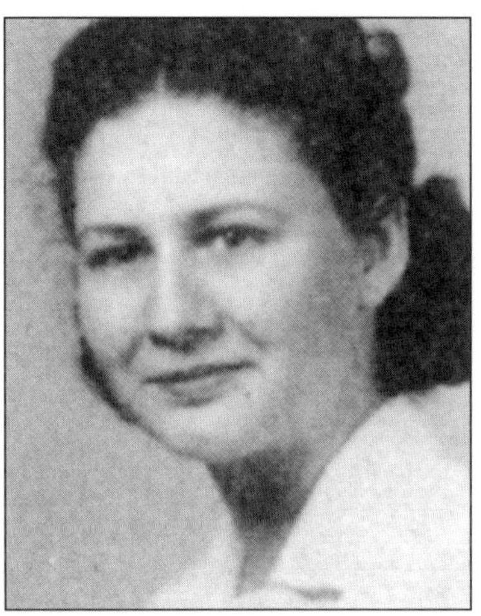

*O*rdella Ida Geisler was born March 4, 1916 in Deshler, Nebraska, a second child for Robert W. and Lydia A. Geisler.

The Geisler family moved to Hebron, Nebraska, when Ordella was eight years old. Robert Geisler was the Sheriff in Hebron, and Lydia a homemaker who stayed busy with Ordella and her four siblings, elder brother Anton, younger sisters Laverna and Ruth, and baby brother Rolland.

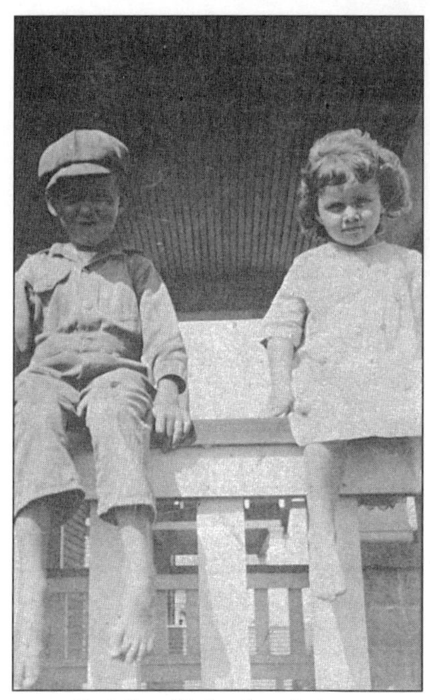
Ordella with brother Anton,
Deshler, Nebraska

Ordella attended Hebron Elementary School, Hebron Academy and Hebron Junior College. In 1940 she transferred to the University of Nebraska.

Ordella was quite certain that a career in veterinary medicine was something she was interested in. Ordella, being a smart young woman, attended night school to attain her pre-veterinary courses. She enjoyed the sciences of which she worked hard at, especially Chemistry.

She spent her days working for Dr. Grant A. Ackerman, at the Lincoln Animal Hospital, with whom she had worked since high school. She loved her work with the animals, and learned first-hand the everyday work of a veterinarian. She learned laboratory tests, assisted with surgery, and being a business like young lady, was receptionist, bookkeeper and stenographer. Her patients appreciated her compassionate and caring manner.

Ordella worked hard to achieve the necessary schooling to get into veterinary school. She was determined to pay her way through College, and even though it took longer than normal, she was able to finish her studies at a slower pace.

It was in 1943, at the age of twenty–seven, that she started looking for veterinary schools to apply to.

She applied to both Iowa State and Kansas State veterinary schools. She asked permission from both schools to send her records and transcript; Iowa State replied simply that they did not accept 'women,' they only accepted men! Kansas State, on the other hand, graciously accepted her! After transferring to Kansas State College in 1943, Ordella received her Bachelor's Degree in Biological Science.

Ordella was admitted to the professional curriculum on May 29, 1944. During World War Two, there were slots that opened up in the professional schools, thus allowing the women to fill them. Because of the effects of World War Two, most colleges, including Kansas State College, went into "accelerated" programs. With permitted completion of training and year round instruction Ordella's class graduated after three years instead of the usual four! This program existed from 1942–1948.

She enjoyed her classmates, of which there were forty-one

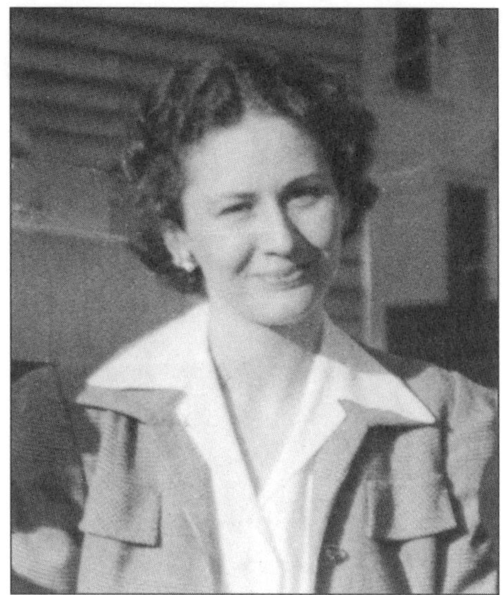

Ordella in 1940

men, and two women. One of the women, Thelma Kanawyer, a good friend was also, a room mate. [Thelma was a war bride, her husband, a veterinarian, ('39 Division of Veterinary Medicine, Kansas State College), was away in the Pacific, in the 1st Calvary Division. Thelma decided to apply to veterinary school and was admitted to the professional curriculum May 29, 1944. She was in her junior year of veterinary school when her husband returned to the states. He was ready to start a practice, so Thelma quit veterinary school to become a housewife, assistant and bookkeeper to her husband.] Thelma remembers Ordella as a 'great gal.'

Ordella and Thelma were joined by a third lady, Ruth Kaslow. Ruth was an older lady from New York who had a previous degree in medical technology.

Ordella remembers that in the summer, days were long, hot and horrible without air-conditioning. She spent probably twenty-seven hours a week in lab work, with additional class work on top of that! Ordella found classes such as Anatomy and Histopathology challenging because of the 'new vocabulary' she had to learn. She felt this was the primary adjustment of her days in veterinary school. Nevertheless, it was an adjustment she enjoyed, as she was always intrigued by new words!

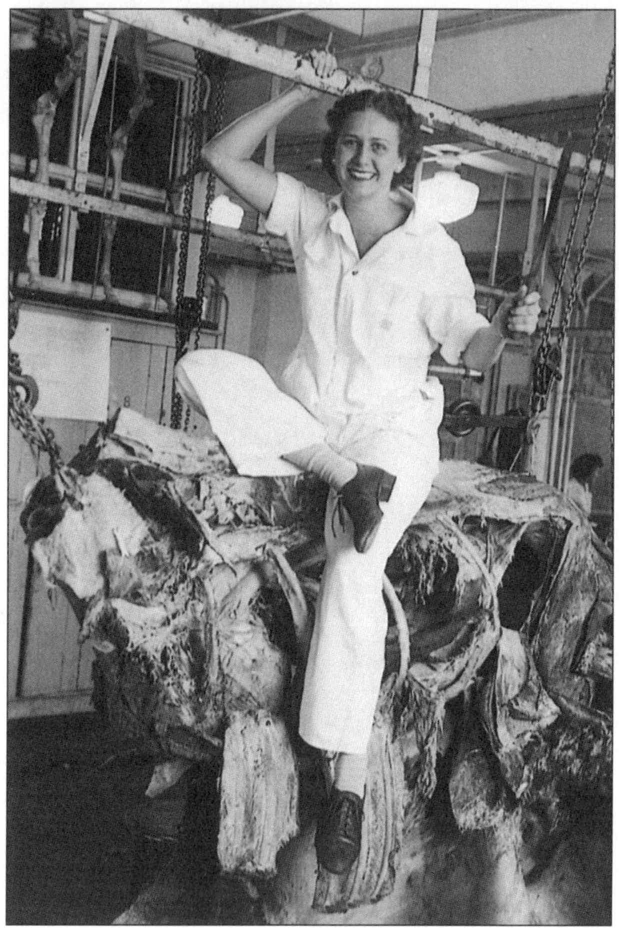

Ordella in the Necropsy Dept.

Ordella enjoyed her class members, and most of her professors, although she remembers the teacher who thought she was wasting her time and she would never repay the tax payers! He would change his mind in later years as many men with the same opinion did!

In general, Ordella's days were fun; the men and women in her class were good sports and good friends. Dr. Gabriel Nossov, a class mate, remembers Ordella, as "A friendly, supportive, and good person."

Any spare time Ordella had was spent working — no campus life as we know it today. She held down a few jobs, keeping books at a local filling station three afternoons, supervised Teen Town for the Kiwanis Club on Friday and Saturday evenings, worked in the veterinary school pharmacy, and graded papers for Dr. Frick (head of the Surgery and Medicine Department).

Another good friend and room mate of Ordella's, Maxine Caley, (assistant to Dean Dykstra and Dean Leasure) attests to the great determination Ordella had to achieve her veterinary degree.

It was in February of 1947 that the degree of Veterinary Medicine was proudly conferred on Dr. Ordella Geisler, alongside forty-one men and one woman.

It was a good time to be a graduate veterinarian, the demand for such professionals was great. Ordella was ready to start her new career.

Following her graduation Dr. Geisler returned to Lincoln, Nebraska, where she joined Dr. Grant Ackerman, in the veterinary hospital that inspired her to become a veterinarian.

Dr. Ordella Geisler was proud of her new degree, and honored to be the first female licensed to practice veterinary medicine in Nebraska.

Ordella, familiar with her surroundings, fell into the daily routine quickly, each new day offering a new challenge. Being a mixed-animal practice, many species were to become Ordella's patients. She remembers one of the more difficult cases that she enjoyed working on, 'snakes with foul mouth,' and removing ticks from the scales of the snake!

Ordella's days reminisced her school days, they were long and tiring, but she loved her work. She worked hard to please her patients and their owners. Not having modern day anesthetics and tranquilizers made every job a little harder. Horses needing surgery were kept docile with ether and chloral hydrate for anesthetic.

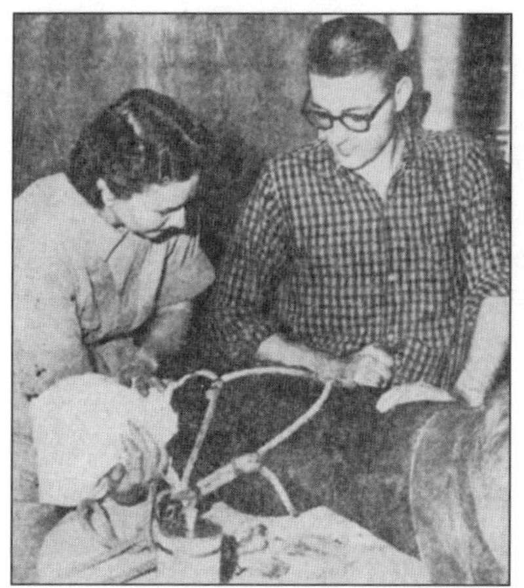

Ordella anesthetizing a horse

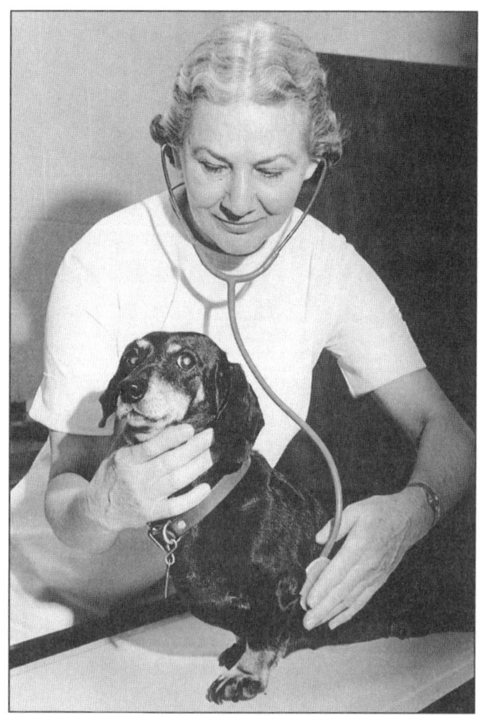

Dr. Ordella Geisler, examining a patient

Everyday the door would open with a new case for Ordella, from marmosets, cats, dogs and a Cardinal with broken leg, and even Kangaroo's! (The Pioneers Park, in Lincoln, Nebraska, kangaroo suffered with frostbitten ears and needed treatment)! Ordella never knew what her next patient would be, but was always ready with a smile!

Ordella enjoyed learning new surgical techniques, always keeping the practice in line with the rigid requirements set forth by the Small Animal Hospital Association. It was quite an achievement in the 1950's to have a full-service animal hospital, with operating rooms and large and small animal treatment areas!

Ordella practiced with Dr. Grant Ackerman, and his son Dr. Ed Ackerman who had joined the practice after his graduation in 1955 from the School of Veterinary Medicine, at Kansas State College. Ordella worked for about twelve years as an associate, before becoming a partner. It was in 1972 that she purchased the hospital from Dr.'s Ackerman, and established her own animal hospital, 'Geisler Animal Hospital.'

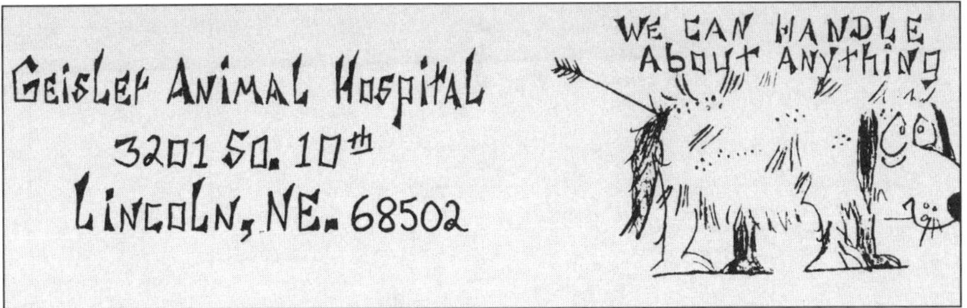

The hospital's letterhead!

Even though the days were long, Ordella never refused help to a sick animal. She was always intrigued at what case the next telephone call would bring her. Her great wit and sense of humor saw her through whenever the need arose.

She recalls the Saturday evening when she was still doing large animal work; a client had called and had a cow with milk fever. On arriving at the farm, the farmer was shocked to see a *lady veterinarian,* and proceeded to tell Ordella what a poor excuse for a veterinarian she was! Of course, Ordella being *'the lady,'* that she is, informed the farmer that she did not know how he was going to do better on a Saturday evening! The cow was treated quite successfully, and the farmer enjoyed Ordella's presence every bit as well as her male counterparts from that day on!

During Ordella's practicing years she was an active member in the Nebraska Veterinary Medical Association. She served as secretary – treasurer from 1950 – 1952, and again in 1959 – 1960. She was also an active member of the American Veterinary Association, and The Association for Women Veterinarians.

Ordella, as dedicated as she was to her animal hospital, took a short break to marry Wendell L. Hoffman, on April 15, 1978!

After practicing for thirty – five years, Ordella retired in 1983. She has spent her retirement years traveling, cooking, sewing, reading and attending class re-unions.

Ordella loves to reminisce about her days working in veterinary practice. She is proud to be a veterinarian, and feels women have come along way and will continue to do so.

Dr. Ordella Geisler is truly a compassionate, caring lady who significantly, through her years of dedication and pure hard work, smoothed a more pleasant path for those who have followed her in the veterinary profession!

Ordella Ida Geisler, D.V.M.
Chronology

1916: 4 March, born in Deshler, Nebraska, to Robert W. and Lydia A. Geisler.

1935: Graduated from Hebron Academy, Hebron, Nebraska

1940: Transferred to the University of Nebraska

1944: 29 May, admitted to the professional curriculum

1946: Secretary of Junior AVMA –second semester officer

1947: 4 February, graduated with the spring class of 1947
Joined Dr. Ackerman, in practice in Lincoln, Nebraska.

1947: Chairman of the Committee on Registration and Information of the
Nebraska State Veterinary Medical Association.

*1950–
1952*: Served as secretary – treasurer of the Nebraska Veterinary Medical
Association.

*1959–
1960*: Secretary – treasurer of the Nebraska Veterinary Medical Association.

1972: Established Geisler Animal Hospital

1978 : Married Wendell L. Hoffman, Manhattan, Kansas.

1979 : 15 April, married Wendell L. Hoffman, Manhattan, Kansas.
Selected for Groundbreakers (an organization for women who have
pioneered in various business and professional fields).

1983 : Retired from active veterinary practice.

Chapter 6

Ruth Kaslow
–1947 School of Veterinary Medicine
Kansas State College

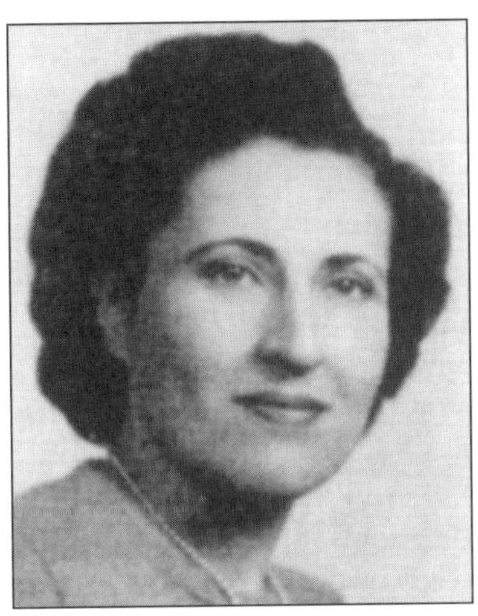

$\mathcal{R}$uth Kaslow was born in Brooklyn, New York, June 26, 1914 to Nathan and Bessie "Berg" Kaslow. Ruth was the first child born to this union.

Growing up in Brooklyn, a borough of New York City was an exciting time for Ruth and her younger brothers Milton and Ted. They enjoyed going to New York City to the movies and museums and, of course to The New York Public Library. As Ruth grew older she enjoyed going out on dinner "dates" and attending the theatre.

Ruth graduated from New Utrecht High School, in Brooklyn in 1931. She loved history and entered Brooklyn College, as a History major.

Ruth's first year in college she was required to take biology. In her first semester of biology she was introduced to Botany, this was interesting to her; but it was in her second semester that she was introduced to Zoology, this fascinated her. After dissecting a Bull frog, a whole new world opened for Ruth. She changed her major to Biology and added a minor in Psychology.

It was during her course of study that Ruth found out about a career as a Medical Lab Technician, a field she entered, upon her graduation from college on February 1, 1935.

Ruth's first job in a small private hospital was as laboratory technician trainee. She was given two meals a day in the staff dining room for her salary. She worked hard and learned all she could, even staying in the evening to practice blood counts and Bacteriology. For her hard work she was rewarded with a paying job when a technician left. After about six months the hospital closed its doors, a disappointment for Ruth as she had become one of the lead technicians. Not deterred, Ruth soon found employment at Brooklyn Jewish Hospital, as a lab tech.

Ruth, who was born with hearing problems and deformities to her fingers (stemming from her mother being exposed early in pregnancy to German measles), had a bright outlook on life.

Ruth came to the attention of Dr. Tarlov, a neurosurgeon who was doing research work on dogs. She worked full-time under his grant. Her work entailed some post-operative animal care of which she enjoyed.

Ruth, who was very conscientious about the care of the animals, realized the importance they had on the experiments.

Ruth's love for animals developed greatly during this time. She found herself wanting to further her education and find out more about them.

Ruth applied to a few veterinary schools, she was happy when Kansas State College wanting to fill the empty seats that the men who were away at war would have had, graciously accepted her. She was admitted to the professional curriculum May 29, 1944.

Ruth felt that veterinary school was a 'wonder,' always having something new to learn. Being an older student she enjoyed the challenge of returning to learning and studying.

Ruth stayed true to her Jewish beliefs, attending worship services at the Hillel Foundation, which was fairly new to the Kansas State campus. She attended weekly discussions of current affairs and participated in debates. The Foundation was honored to have the college president, President Milton Eisenhower, attend their first Passover celebration (Seder Meal).

Ruth's hearing loss became more extensive in her early twenties, so

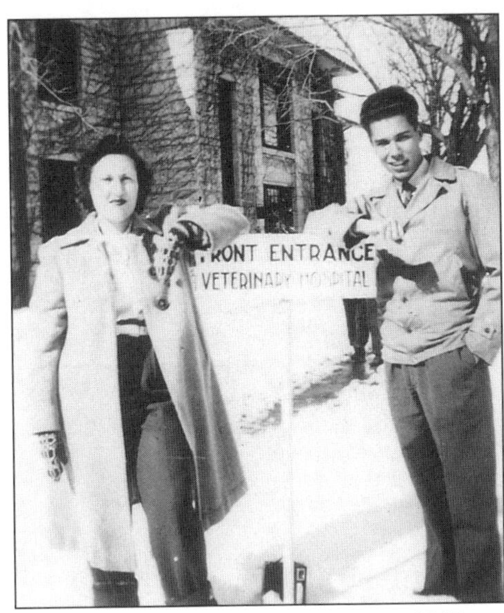

Ruth and Gabe Nossov, KSCSVM, 1945

she wore hearing aids. Sadly, in veterinary school her hearing loss became greater and the hearing aids were of no use. Ruth learned to lip-read and became a 'cracker-jack' at doing so. She trained her pet cat to wake her in the morning when her alarm went off, so as she would not be late for school.

Ruth loved her classes and enjoyed the help of Dr. W. M. McLeod, who she remembers as 'a very special guy.' She also was thankful for the friendship of Dr. Folse who was a good instructor.

Ruth became a good friend and 'motherly figure' to many of the 'boys' from back East. She remembers Gabe Nossov as an especially fine 'guy.'

Some of the young men shared common ground with Ruth, they were minorities. Some were Hispanic, some Jewish, some African-American. Ruth was Jewish, female and had deformities! It was not always a good time for Ruth. She remembered reading the lips of many a person (students and professors alike) who 'vilified' her. Ruth was proud that President Eisenhower (college president) was part of an effort to change such attitudes. Ruth held her head high and moved on!

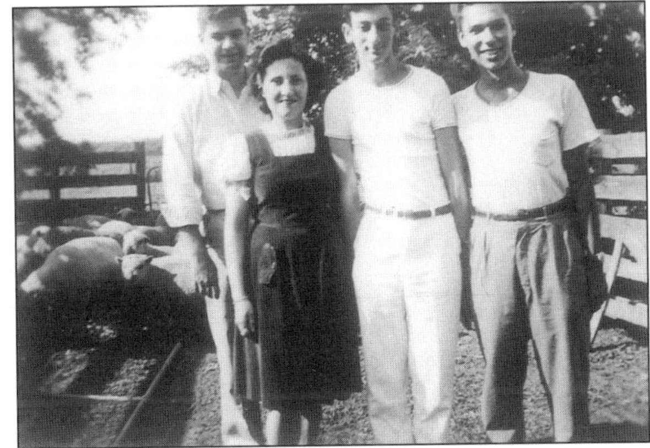

Ruth and classmates, July 1944

Ruth, being in the accelerated program, worked year round to complete all her required classes in three years, instead of the usual four.

She proudly accepted her veterinary degree, alongside one other female and forty one men, on February 4, 1947. Ruth was also proud to be elected and initiated as a member of the all college honor society Phi Kappa Phi (a national honorary scholastic fraternity for men and women, based on high scholarship and character).

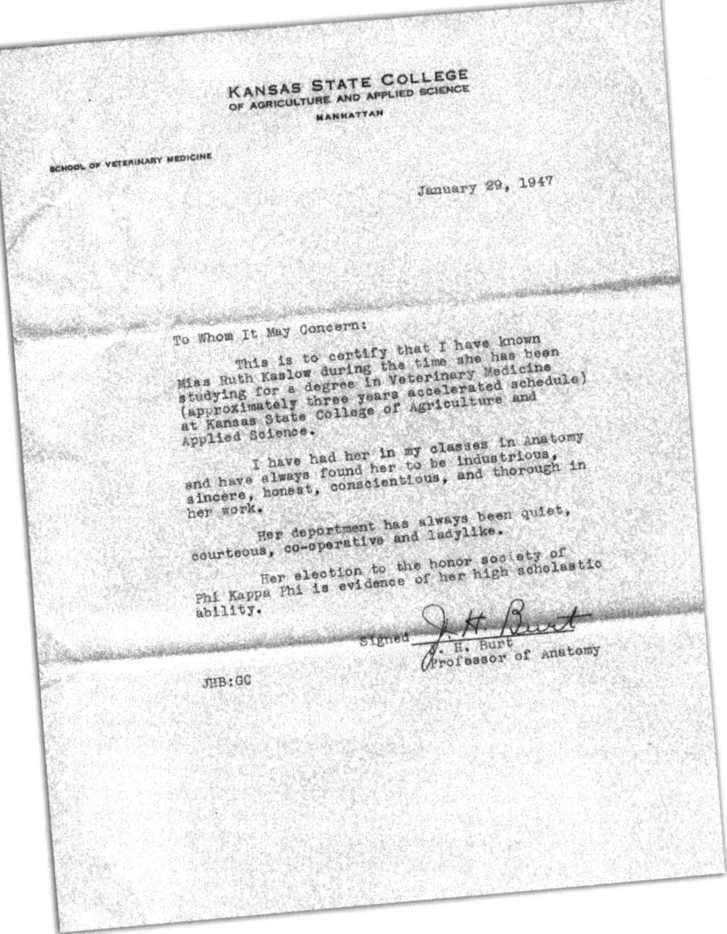

KANSAS STATE COLLEGE
OF AGRICULTURE AND APPLIED SCIENCE
MANHATTAN

SCHOOL OF VETERINARY MEDICINE

January 29, 1947

To Whom It May Concern:

This is to certify that I have known Miss Ruth Kaslow during the time she has been studying for a degree in Veterinary Medicine (approximately three years accelerated schedule) at Kansas State College of Agriculture and Applied Science.

I have had her in my classes in Anatomy and have always found her to be industrious, sincere, honest, conscientious, and thorough in her work.

Her deportment has always been quiet, courteous, co-operative and ladylike.

Her election to the honor society of Phi Kappa Phi is evidence of her high scholastic ability.

Signed J. H. Burt
J. H. Burt
Professor of Anatomy

JHB:GC

Letters of Recommendation, from Dr's Dykstra and Burt

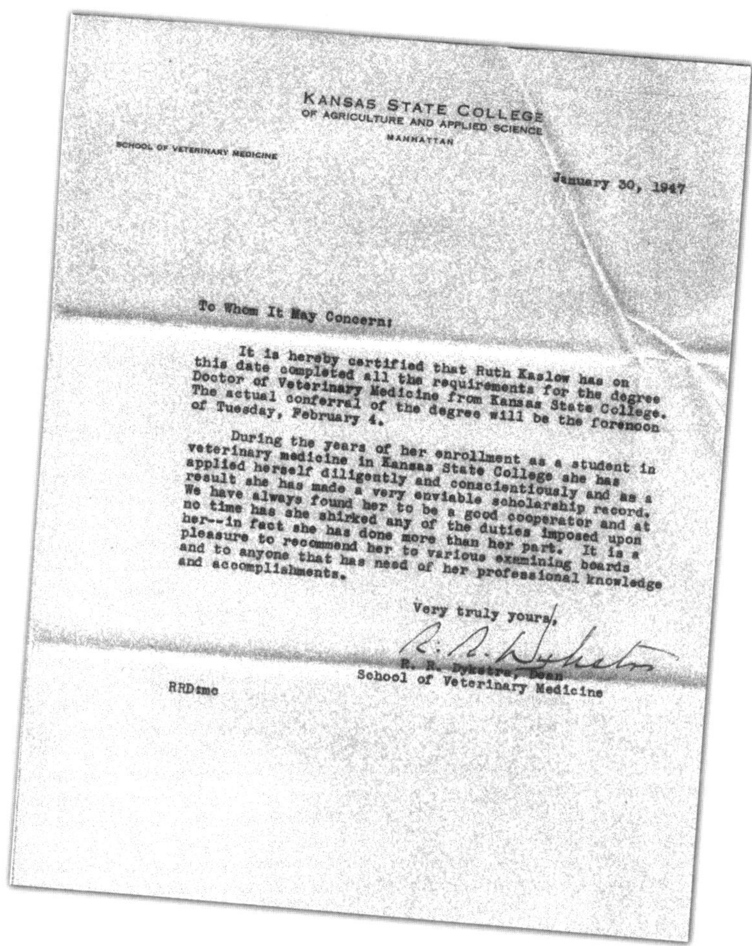

Letters of Recommendation, from Dr's Dykstra and Burt

Dr. Ruth Kaslow returned to New York, where she worked full-time at the Brooklyn Jewish Hospital. She was honored to be the Research Technician in charge of the animal research department. She worked long hours taking care of and improving the conditions of the animals in this department.

Ruth took time out to marry Murray Zaret, on June 20, 1948. During their marriage, Murray opened the Coney Island Petting Zoo, where he strived to familiarize children and their families with a variety of animals ranging from goats, dogs and cats to snakes and spiders! In the sixties Murray and his animals were frequent guests on "The Beachcomber Bill Show," a New York TV show for children.

Dr. Kaslow, as she chose to be called through her professional career, was sought after by the doctors at the hospital, and despite her lack of hearing she knew emphatically what they needed. Ruth, from experience, was able to tell from the surgeons eyes and hands what she needed to do for them.

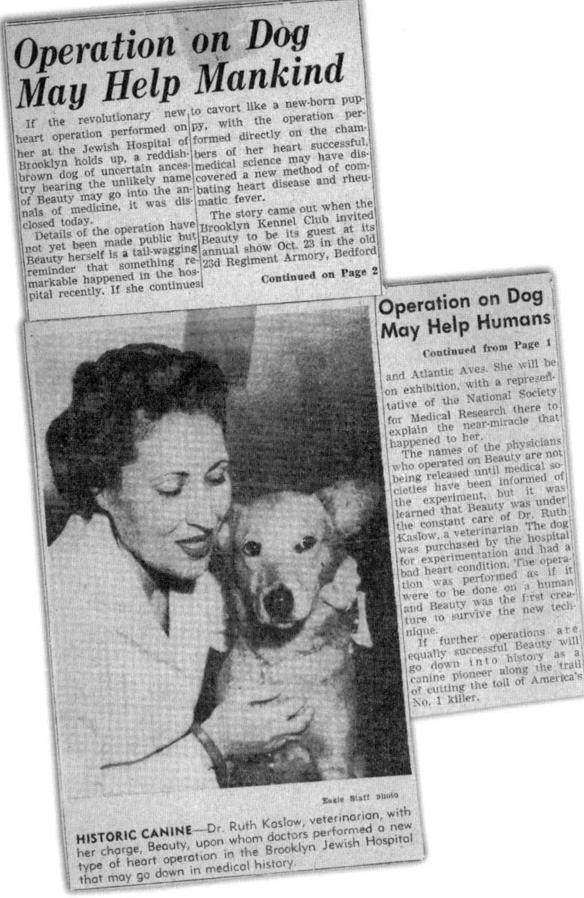

Operation on Dog May Help Mankind

If the revolutionary new heart operation performed on her at the Jewish Hospital of Brooklyn holds up, a reddish-brown dog of uncertain ancestry bearing the unlikely name of Beauty may go into the annals of medicine, it was disclosed today.

Details of the operation have not yet been made public but Beauty herself is a tail-wagging reminder that something remarkable happened in the hospital recently. If she continues to cavort like a new-born puppy, with the operation performed directly on the chambers of her heart successful, medical science may have discovered a new method of combating heart disease and rheumatic fever.

The story came out when the Brooklyn Kennel Club invited Beauty to be its guest at its annual show Oct. 23 in the old 23d Regiment Armory, Bedford

Continued on Page 2

Operation on Dog May Help Humans

Continued from Page 1

and Atlantic Aves. She will be on exhibition, with a representative of the National Society for Medical Research there to explain the near-miracle that happened to her.

The names of the physicians who operated on Beauty are not being released until medical societies have been informed of the experiment, but it was learned that Beauty was under the constant care of Dr. Ruth Kaslow, a veterinarian. The dog was purchased by the hospital for experimentation and had a bad heart condition. The operation was performed as if it were to be done on a human and Beauty was the first creature to survive the new technique.

If further operations are equally successful Beauty will go down into history as a canine pioneer along the trail of cutting the toll of America's No. 1 killer.

Eagle Staff Photo

HISTORIC CANINE—Dr. Ruth Kaslow, veterinarian, with her charge, Beauty, upon whom doctors performed a new type of heart operation in the Brooklyn Jewish Hospital that may go down in medical history.

Ruth found her work more fascinating than ever. It was the beginning of many medical research advancements, vascular grafts and open heart surgery that topped the list.

Ruth, along with five medical doctors, authored a paper entitled _The Use of Antiperistaltic Bowel Segments Following Massive Small Bowel Resection_. It was an exciting time for Ruth, she was proud to be a part of it!

Ruth was an active member of the AVMA (American Veterinary Medical Association), and N.Y. and N.Y.C. veterinary associations.

Ruth's professional accomplishments did not go unnoticed. In 1966 The Animal Welfare Institute of New York City, gave the Jewish Hospital of Brooklyn, one of two top ratings for animal care. Dr. Ruth Kaslow was cited for outstanding care of laboratory animals used for scientific research.

Ruth loved her work and devoted her time to the betterment of living conditions for animals. She was proud to show off the animals and their living conditions to anyone who so wished. She realized that the environment the animals lived in was important to their well-being; she invented or borrowed equipment to make it as comfortable as possible.

Her love and commitment towards the care of the animals was honored with WARDS (Working for Animals used in Research Drugs and Surgery) first Animal Handling and Housing Award. Ruth was proud to demonstrate that professional care can be enforced, if research administration and scientists appreciate well cared for animals!

WARDS Awards Dr. Kaslow For A Pain and Stress Saving System

Dr. Ruth Kaslow has received WARDS first Animal Handling and Housing Award because she has invented or borrowed so many ways to lessen the stress and suffering of her animals used in research. She has proved that even in a sub-basement of a crowded urban area professional care is possible. She has exploded the myth that tight caging is necessary or desirable.

The first difference in her laboratory, at the Jewish Hospital in Brooklyn, is that she says to "come right over" and see it. There is no delay while the mess is cleaned up. If there is any disorder she can explain it to an unexpected visitor like any good doctor could make a waiting room full of patients understand an emergency case.

The new animal is put in a pen in which wood shavings are treated with flea killer. It is given food and water and left to rest. Her dogs are not debarked (the vocal cords cut). Next day most of the dogs are able to be handled because they have friendly surroundings. How different from the wholesale process where dog is debarked, put in a dip for fleas and left to shiver in a grid bottom small cage.

All dogs are kept in pens by Dr. Kaslow. Workers with brooms clean out the shavings. These dogs are not afraid. On the theory that a calm, trustful animal is the best for research Dr. Kaslow produces this kind of animal.

Dr. Kaslow is on the job at 6 o'clock in the morning. According to her this is the best time to see if any animals are ill. The slow, listless ones can be observed in the roomy pens in a way not possible in a cramped cage.

Before being operated on the animal is given a tranquilizer and then an anaesthetic. Her operating table is designed to minimize the suffering of the animal after surgery. Since the dog must be on its back her stainless steel operating table is fitted with a four inch foam rubber pad that is cut out like a trough. The animal fits into this. This plastic covered base holds the animal in position perfectly and prevents bruises and sores caused by tight trussing on a hard table.

All tubes and other material that must be inserted in the animal during an experiment are the latest soft pain saving kind in use for human surgery. She wants her animal back to normal as soon as possible.

Dr. Kaslow never leaves an animal until it has gained consciousness and she knows the extent to which pain will have to be deadened for an uneventful recovery. The dog is placed for the night in a large cage whose drafty grid bottom is padded with a blanket and sheet. When an animal needs to be nursed back she has a shelf full of good food to tempt its appetite.

Dr. Kaslow has proved that professional care can be set up anywhere if the research administration and the scientists appreciate well cared for animals and there is dedicated leadership in the laboratory.

In our next leaflet we will have pictures and news about how we will help Dr. Kaslow continue her good work.

In 1967, while working at the Montefiore Hospital, Ruth was asked to work with an architect on a new animal research facility. Ruth was delighted when as an incentive for her expertise; the hospital provided her with a car and driver to take her to and from work. Years later an apartment near to the hospital was provided. Ruth was to have control of the arrangement of the facility, select cages and arrange all aspects of the new facility. This was truly a highlight in her career!

Ruth devoted a good part of her life to her work, her passion being the care of animals. Ruth enjoyed her spare time, gardening, breeding and raising many varieties of tropical fish. She enjoyed spending time with her children, grandchildren and great-grandchildren, until poor health required her to be in a care facility.

Ruth worked hard to have a better understanding of animals. Her knowledge of the care of animals in biologic experimentation has left an indelible mark on the future of animal research.

Ruth loved her work, and enjoyed the people she worked with. She was cited in the ninth edition of Who's Who of American Women, 1975–1976. Many people have benefited from having known Ruth. Her love and care for animals will never be forgotten!

Ruth Kaslow
Chronology

1914: 26, June born Brooklyn, New York, to Nathan and Bess (Berg) Kaslow.

1931: Graduated New Utrecht High School, Brooklyn, New York.

1935: Received B.A. at Brooklyn College, Brooklyn, New York.

1935-1943: Worked in medical lab at Trinity, Jewish Hospitals, Brooklyn, NY.

1944: 29 May, admitted to the Professional Curriculum, Kansas State College, School of Veterinary Medicine.

1947: 4 February, Graduated D.V.M., Kansas State College, School of Veterinary Medicine. Elected and inducted to Phi Kappa Phi.

1947-1967: Veterinarian at Jewish Hospital, Brooklyn, New York

1948: 20 June, married Murray Zaret.

1967: Veterinarian at Montefiore Hospital, and Medical Center, Bronx, New York.

1972 : Retires from active practice, circa.

1975-1976 : Who's Who of American Women, 9th edition.

Chapter 7

Mary Letitia Hammomd
–1947 School of Veterinary Medicine
Kansas State College

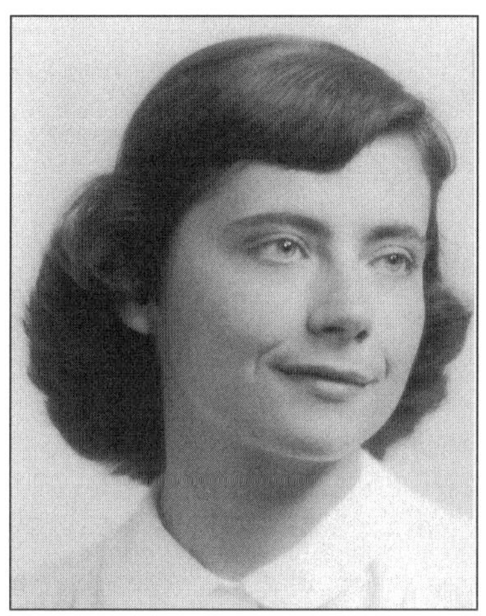

 ary Letitia Hammond, the youngest child and only daughter of Ralph H. Hammond and Yvonne "Bouchard" Hammond, was born on September 14th, 1925, in Cleveland, Ohio.

Ralph was a statistician whose birthplace was Ohio, and Yvonne, a teacher in a private school was from France. Mary and her older brothers Henri and Paul enjoyed spending time visiting France with their mother.

The Hammond children enjoyed their early years growing up in Shaker Heights, Ohio. Their big, three story house was a haven for the active young children and their faithful German shepherd dog "Annie."

When Mary was about six years old, she was lucky to spend the summer with her mother and brothers visiting family in France. It was a glorious summer, sadly marred by a cablegram notifying Yvonne and the children that their home in Shaker Heights had burned down and their beloved father and husband had died in the flames!

It was a sad time for Mary and her family. They were saddened further by the account of the Shaker Heights Sheriff of the fire. A fire had apparently started in the basement of the home, and had spread to a refrigerating unit where, a tank containing the refrigerant liquid blew up. The house soon filled with ammonia fumes. Mr. Hammond who was sleeping on the third floor was suffocated by the fumes, but not before the family dog Annie had pulled him from his bed and dragged him about twenty five feet to the top of the stairs. Annie was lying dead alongside her master. Annie, not able to drag her master any further, had chewed holes through the outer wall of the house. She could have escaped if she had wanted, but chose to stay with her master. She was a great dog!

The next few years in Mary's life were spent in France where she learned to speak French and attained schooling.

Mary, with her mother and brother Paul, returned to America, to live in San Diego, California. Her elder brother Henri stayed back in France with an uncle's family to finish all of his schooling. In later years Henri worked as an interpreter for the League of Nations.

Mary was close to her brother Paul and idolized him. Probably having no father, she depended on brother Paul to take care of her. A job, for the most part, which he took seriously! There was a humorous time, when they lived in France, apparently Mrs. Hammond was to meet her children at a sidewalk café at an appointed time. Mary and Paul waited patiently for their mother, who evidently had been held up somewhere. They swiftly decided to entertain themselves by drinking the remains of all the drinks left at other tables. Their mother eventually arrived to find two quite 'happy' children!

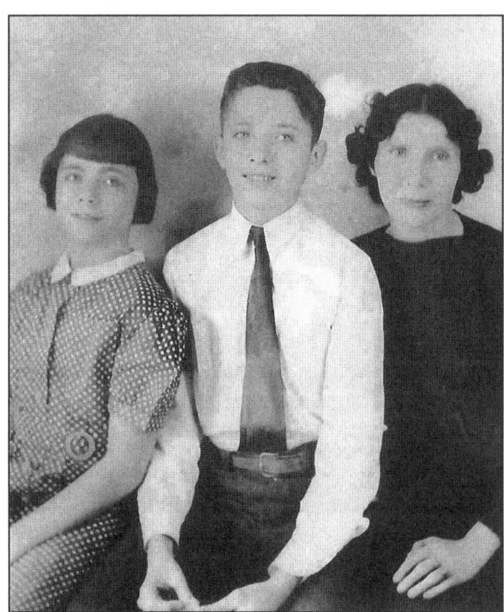

Mary and Paul with their mother Yvonne

Mary shared a great love for animals with her brother Paul, having a menagerie of pets, including dogs, cats, lizards, horses, snakes and tortoises.

It was no shock when first Paul, then Mary, both announced they wanted to become veterinarians!

Paul attended veterinary school at Colorado State University, after which he practiced for three years in a large animal practice. Becoming disillusioned, he returned to Minnesota University and acquired his PhD in Toxicology.

Mary, following in Paul's footsteps, upon graduating from Grossmont Union High School, attended San Diego State College. It was at San Diego, after earning pre-requisites for veterinary school that Mary applied to two veterinary schools.

One of the two colleges accepting women at this time was Kansas State College. Mary was excited to be accepted to their veterinary program.

Mary enjoyed life in veterinary school. Although small in size, she was quite able to take care of herself. She enjoyed her classmates for the most part, finding a good friend Phyllis Hickney the only other female in her class.

Mary worked hard in her studies, sometimes struggling with subjects that required math as this was not a natural subject for her. She was attending school through the war years and being in a class that was in the accelerated program meant that she was able to finish her veterinary degree in three years instead of the usual four.

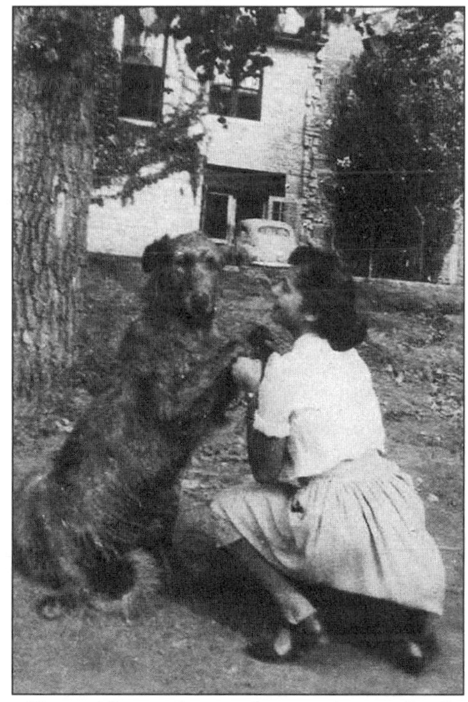

Mary with a patient at the veterinary school

Mary was lucky to have for her lab partner her friend Phyllis. They shared an equine cadaver that they christened "Letitia Mae," both the ladies middle names.

Mary was honored, while in veterinary school, to be elected into Gamma Sigma Delta (a society encouraging high standards of excellence in agricultural and related sciences).

In Mary's junior year the veterinary school was badly damaged by fire. The students and faculty worked hard to clean debris, so that they could continue as best they could with classes. Dirty and exhausted, Mary's classmate Phyllis remembered sitting with her friend against the outside wall of the clinic and smoking a cigarette. For Mary, a smoker, and Phyllis who was smoking for the first and only time in her life, it felt good after all the heavy, hard work!

On June 1, 1947, Mary, alongside her friend Phyllis and twenty-one men, received her degree in veterinary medicine.

Dr. Mary Hammond, after a short trip to Europe, worked temporarily in a small-animal practice in Brooklyn, New York. Mary had also applied for a position at the Wyoming State Veterinary Laboratory, in Laramie. She was happy to be offered the position and started work sometime in the fall of 1947.

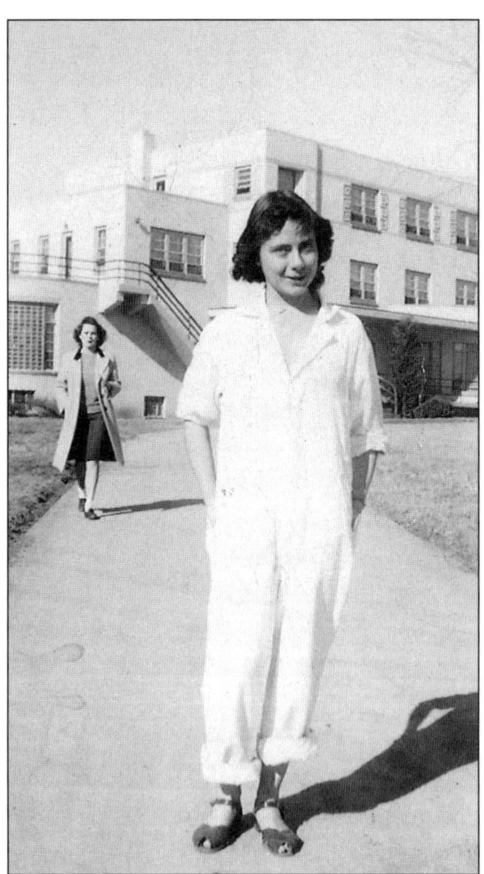

Mary in her first year at veterinary school

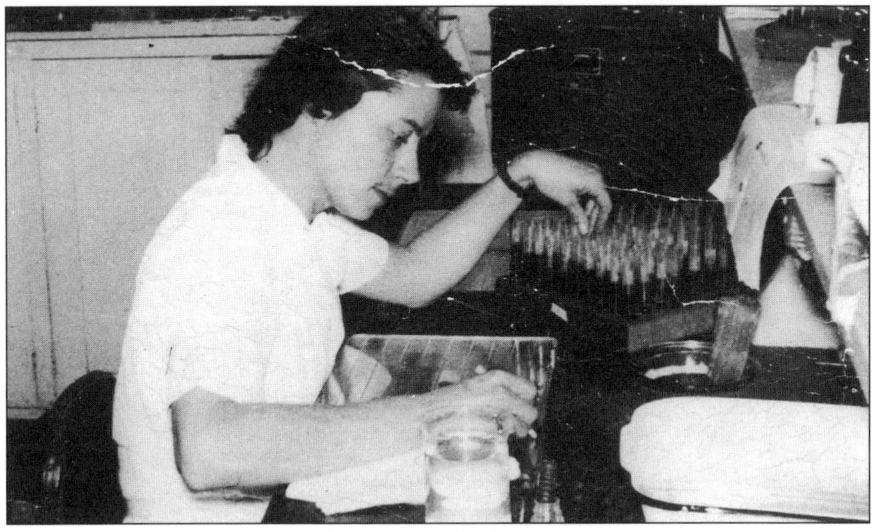

Working hard in the laboratory

In 1948, Mary was united in marriage to John Harvey Glenn, a gentleman she had met at Kansas State. John had been a student in electrical engineering and graduated the same year as Mary.

John, knowing his new brides love for animals, presented her with a pair of Labrador pups as a wedding gift. The pups "Gus" and "Jenny," brought much enjoyment to the newlyweds.

Later in 1948, Mary and John re-located to Santiago in Chile, as John had accepted a position with General Electric. Mary was not able to get a license to practice there, and even if she could have the Chileans thought the whole idea of a woman being a veterinarian was quite preposterous!

After about three years they returned back home. John had apparently felt some latent interest in medicine and being disappointed with his present career, entered

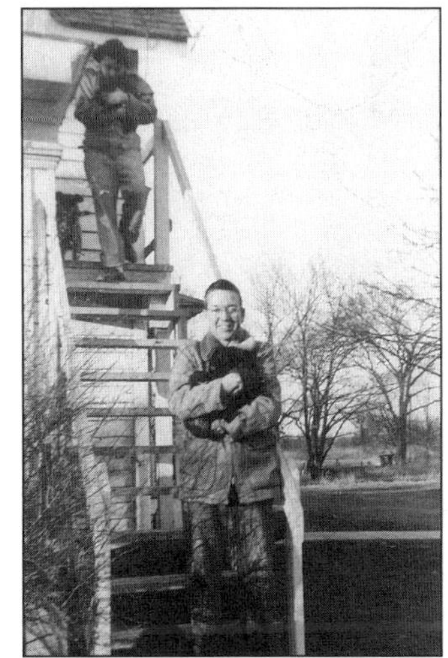

Mary and husband with
their canine family

medical school in about 1952.

Mary took a position at the Illinois State Laboratory, in Centralia, working in the diagnostic laboratory. She worked at the lab for the next few years, putting John through medical school and a residency in pathology. John attended Washington University School of Medicine in St. Louis.

In 1954, Mary and John were blessed with the birth of a son Paul Edward. Young Paul was joined in 1956 by a baby brother, John David, and again in 1957 with another brother, William Cooper. The family was completed in May of 1959, when a baby girl, Ann Odette was born.

Mary had retired from active practice in 1954 when son Paul was born, she was kept with her new baby. She loved her family and enjoyed sharing her French cuisine, spoiling them with pastries, crepes, croissants and baba au rhum. Mary's son John remembers that chicken was never eaten in their house. Mary's work in diagnostic laboratories had evidently left her with a life-long dread and hatred of the bird! Mary also enjoyed her garden, producing fruits and spectacular roses.

Mary became veterinarian to the neighborhood kids' pets. The children knew where to take their sick or injured animals to be cared for.

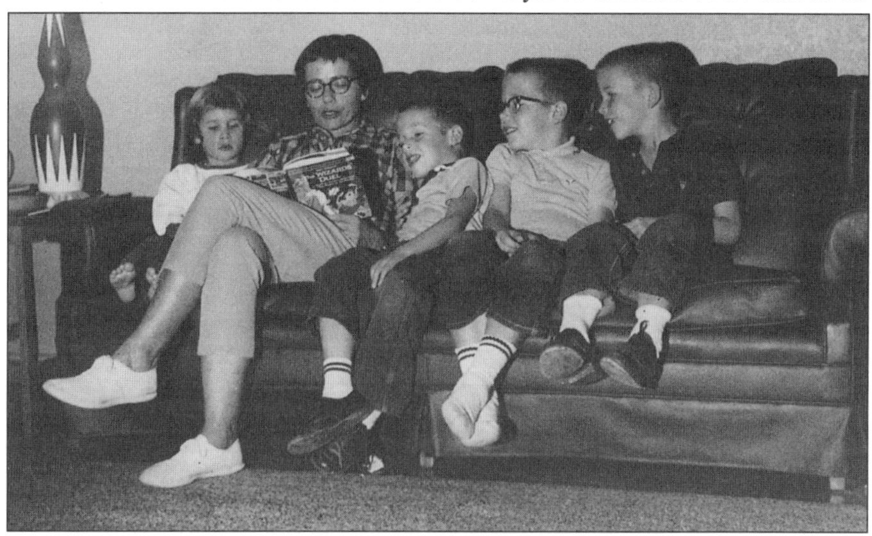

Mary reading to her children, circa 1963

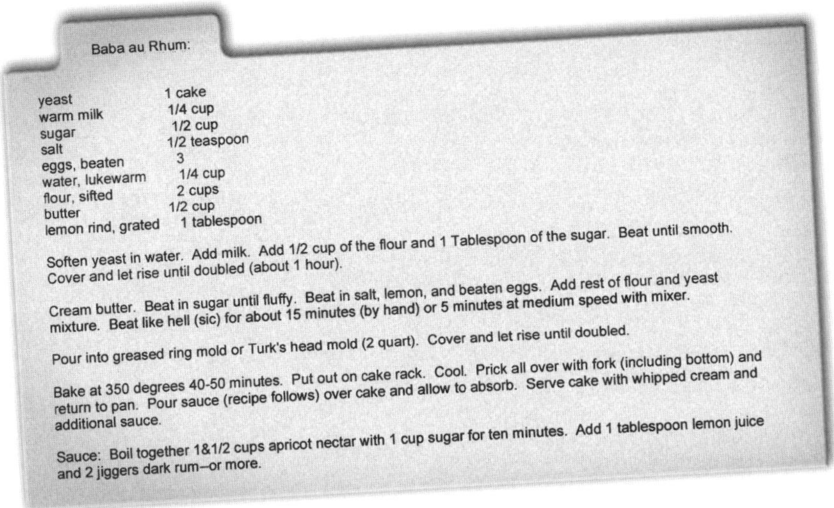

A favorite recipe of Mary's

Daughter Ann remembers when her best friend's Guinea pig had got its leg hung up in its cage and broke it. Mary fashioned the little animal a special splint, and in time he healed just fine.

Son Paul remembers the special care his mother took of their pets, and that one or more of the animals worshiped her above all other people.

Mary and John spent their retirement years in Las Cruces, New Mexico. Mary loved being of service and enjoyed working for 'Literacy Volunteers,' teaching inmates at the prison in Las Cruces to read.

Dr. Mary "Hammond" Glenn achieved a position in veterinary medicine that at the time was not considered a place for women. Nevertheless, she did. Even though she only practiced for a short while, she did a great job and loved it!

Mary passed away October 8, 1995.

THE LADY IS A VETERINARIAN

Mary Letitia Hammond
Chronology

1925 : 14 September, born in Cleveland, Ohio.

1943 : Graduated from Grossmont Union High School, California.
Attended San Diego State College.

1944 : 26 September, admitted to professional curriculum, Kansas State College, School of Veterinary Medicine.

1947 : June, Graduated from veterinary school.
Worked temporarily for a veterinarian in New York.
Started work at Wyoming State Veterinary Laboratory, Laramie, Wyoming.

1948 : Married James Harvey Glenn

1954 : Retired from active practice.
28 October, son Paul Edward Glenn born.

1956 : 22 June, son John David born.

1957 : 17 September, son William Cooper born.

1959 : 16 May, daughter Ann Odette born.

1995 : 8 October, passed away in Las Cruces, New Mexico.

Chapter 8

Phyllis Mae Hickney
–1947 School of Veterinary Medicine
Kansas State College

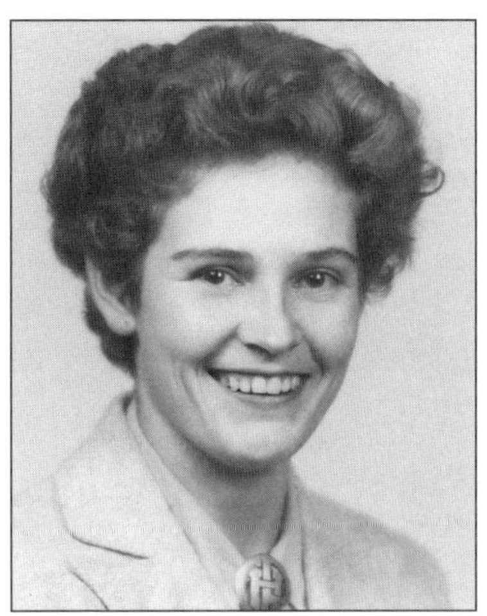

Phyllis Mae Hickney was born on March 26, 1923, to Augustus James Hickney and Marion "Davis" Hickney. Phyllis was the third daughter and fourth child born to this union.

The young Phyllis was well taken care of, having sisters Zoë, and Keitha, and a brother Reginald, who were all ten to thirteen years older than her. She was happy to have a younger brother, Leon, arrive four years after her to complete the Hickney family. By the time Phyllis was eight years old all but Leon had left home.

Maybe it was the times Phyllis spent at the dairy farms that her father Augustus managed in Massachusetts, or maybe from genes of farming ancestors, that she acquired her love for animals.

Phyllis enjoyed watching her father and the herdsmen take care of the dairy cows, observing and taking a mental note of all they were doing. It was not unusual to see Phyllis helping the herdsmen feed the cows their beet pulp. She loved to see the cows happy; at five or six years of age she considered them to be her friends!

Phyllis made many wonderful adult acquaintances as a young child, ones that she remembered for life. They were to leave a lasting impression on the always 'thinking' young Phyllis.

One person that left his mark on her way of thinking was the State Veterinarian, Dr. Thayer. Phyllis watched closely as he tested the dairy cows for tuberculosis, sometimes his testing was favorable and sometimes not. The cows that were positive were sent on their way. Phyllis's mother told her that Phyllis had always wanted to know how Dr. Thayer knew whether or not the cows were to be sent away! She was upset when they left and wanted to know why!

Phyllis enjoyed her school years; she liked everybody, but didn't require close friends to be happy. Growing up, she considered the dogs, cats, rabbits, guinea pigs and farm animals to be her playmates.

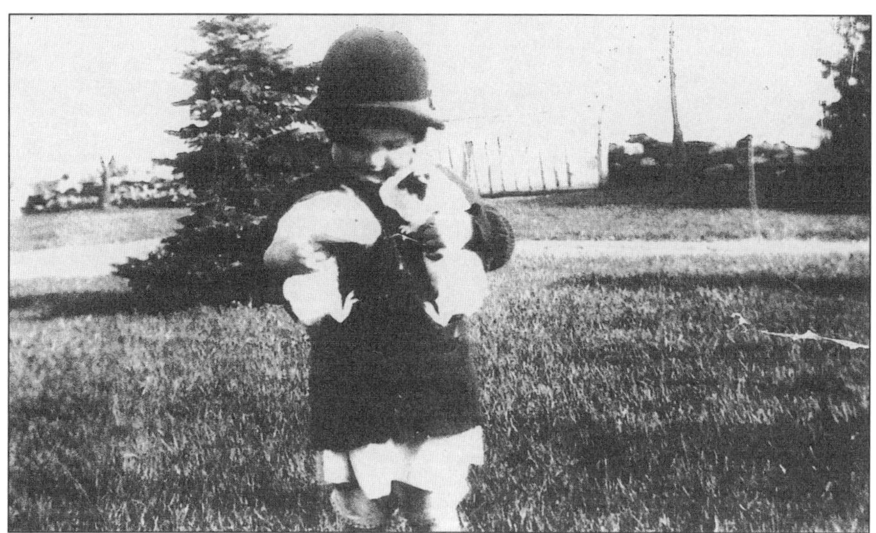

Phyllis on the farm in Massachusetts, with her friends the guinea pigs, circa 1925

She loved to read and felt quite at home in libraries, reading Nancy Drew, Girl Detective and Earl Derr Biggers' Charlie Chan mysteries. Phyllis's other hobbies included stamp collecting and writing poems. Poetry was a way she could express the way she felt about the many things in life that she enjoyed, disliked or had something to say about!

When Phyllis was in eighth grade she became a girl scout, here she was able to experience new and exciting challenges. This was an organization that she championed for many years.

Due to her father managing different farms in Massachusetts, Phyllis attended a few elementary and junior high schools, spending two years at a high school in Dartmouth, Massachusetts, transferring her final two years to David Prouty , High School, in Spencer, Massachusetts. The principal here was a gentleman that Phyllis held with high regard. Likewise, Mr. Agard the school superintendent and principal thought a lot of Phyllis.

At Prouty, Phyllis participated on the debate team and almost became a die-hard baseball fan!

Phyllis graduated from high school in 1940, with a tuition scholarship, including room and board to the prestigious Vassar College in the scenic Hudson Valley, north of New York City, in a town called Poughkeepsie. Phyllis was proud to have persuaded the school superintendent to let her give the valedictory speech on stamp collecting as a hobby!

At Vassar, Phyllis stayed busy. When she was not in classes she spent time doing extra-curricular activities through the non-denominational campus church. She chaired work projects in poor communities in Poughkeepsie, and was founder of the race relations group. She attended lectures outside her own classes, entering into lengthy discussions. With the world at war, she had much to discuss. Phyllis, even though believing in a representative government, also believed that war was not the way to solve problems. She took solace in thought, whilst walking in the woods and feeding the campus squirrels.

While studying zoology at Vassar, it occurred to Phyllis that veterinary medicine might be the place to pursue her growing interest in the comparative structure and function of animals. In the summer of 1943, she worked on a general farm in Connecticut, gaining experience with a wide variety of animals. She occasionally rode along with a mixed – animal practitioner that she described as being "Old, but up-to-date".

It was a fun summer, bringing back happy memories of her childhood back on the farms in Massachusetts.

Phyllis applied to three veterinary colleges, Iowa State, Washington State and Kansas State. Iowa State replied "No women." Washington State and Kansas State said, "Come."

Which veterinary school to attend was decided by mere fate. Phyllis's brother-in-law was a Calvary officer serving under Patton and had been sent to Fort Riley in Manhattan, Kansas when he came down with malaria. Sister Zoë and her husband, by the fall of 1944, were living on Poyntz Avenue in Manhattan. They offered Phyllis a free place to live, with breakfast and dinner.

Phyllis graduated from Vassar College in April, 1944, with an A.B. in Zoology. She felt that her record was respectable, even though she struggled a little with chemistry in her second year. She was proud to leave Vassar as the only 'Danforth Special Student Fellow' ever.

Phyllis was admitted to the professional curriculum at Kansas State College, School of Veterinary Medicine, on September 26, 1944. She entered during the war years, which meant that she entered into the accelerated program, which held classes year round. On completion of all the required classes she would graduate after three years instead of the usual four.

Phyllis liked having her big sister around. Zoë became a sounding board for Phyllis's lectures that she gave after expanding her knowledge of comparative anatomy. She was happy living with them for a year, after which they moved away.

At K-State, Phyllis threw herself into studying, working and of course, extra-curricular causes. One such cause was when she met with the College's President, Milton S. Eisenhower. Phyllis wanted to help a friend from her undergraduate class at Vassar. The friend, a teacher at a Japanese relocation Center in California, had a student she thought might be suited to Kansas State College. Phyllis enquired to the Director of Admissions who informed her that no Japanese could be admitted to any Kansas Educational Institution that was funded by public monies.

Phyllis, not accepting this, conferred with Milton S. Eisenhower. In short, even though Phyllis did not help her friend's student, she felt proud to know the College's President and understand his goals. One of those goals was to do away with the onerous rule about Japanese people not being able to attend Kansas State.

One of Phyllis's jobs was working in the Reading Room, (Library) a job she loved. She enjoyed discussing with Dean R. Dykstra, her employer, how to file the cards, what new books to order and how often to drill holes in the batch of issues of the journals (The drill was the one that Dr. Max McLeod used for wiring big bones to be used for skeletons).

Phyllis, like many students, was asked by Dean Dykstra to sign a promissory note to say they would contribute to the reading room after graduation. He would follow-up with reminders should the students not come through with their commitments.

Phyllis was happy to have an occasion even before she left veterinary school to help the reading room.

It happened after Dr. E. R. Frank had rendered services to a young Hereford bull. The owner of the bull was happy to know that after a little surgery, the bull would be sound for breeding. The owner asked Phyllis what the charge was for the service rendered (no fees were charged at this time for the knowledge or skill of a college clinician). Dr. Frank, who was now working on a horse, looked over his shoulder and answered, "About fifty cents." The owner of the bull, who now realized his animal, was worth far more to him than when he came into the veterinary school, thought fifty cents was not enough. The quick thinking Phyllis explained that they could only charge for drugs and supplies, adding that if he would like to, he could contribute to the Veterinary Reading Room to show his appreciation!

Phyllis shared the antics of the everyday classes with her friend Mary Hammond, the only other girl in their class.

Being one of two females in a class of twenty-one men meant, even for the attractive Phyllis, that the odds were against the women. One day though, the tables turned on the men. It was on ambulatory duty to a farm owned by Dan Casement, the well-to-do son of the famous chief construction engineer of the Union Pacific Railroad that Phyllis was the minority singled out! Upon arriving at the farm where there were Hereford cattle, it was noticeable to the clinician and students that the owner and a couple of hands were having a degree of difficulty in getting a calf to suck a bottle. Phyllis remembers Mr. Casement who had spied

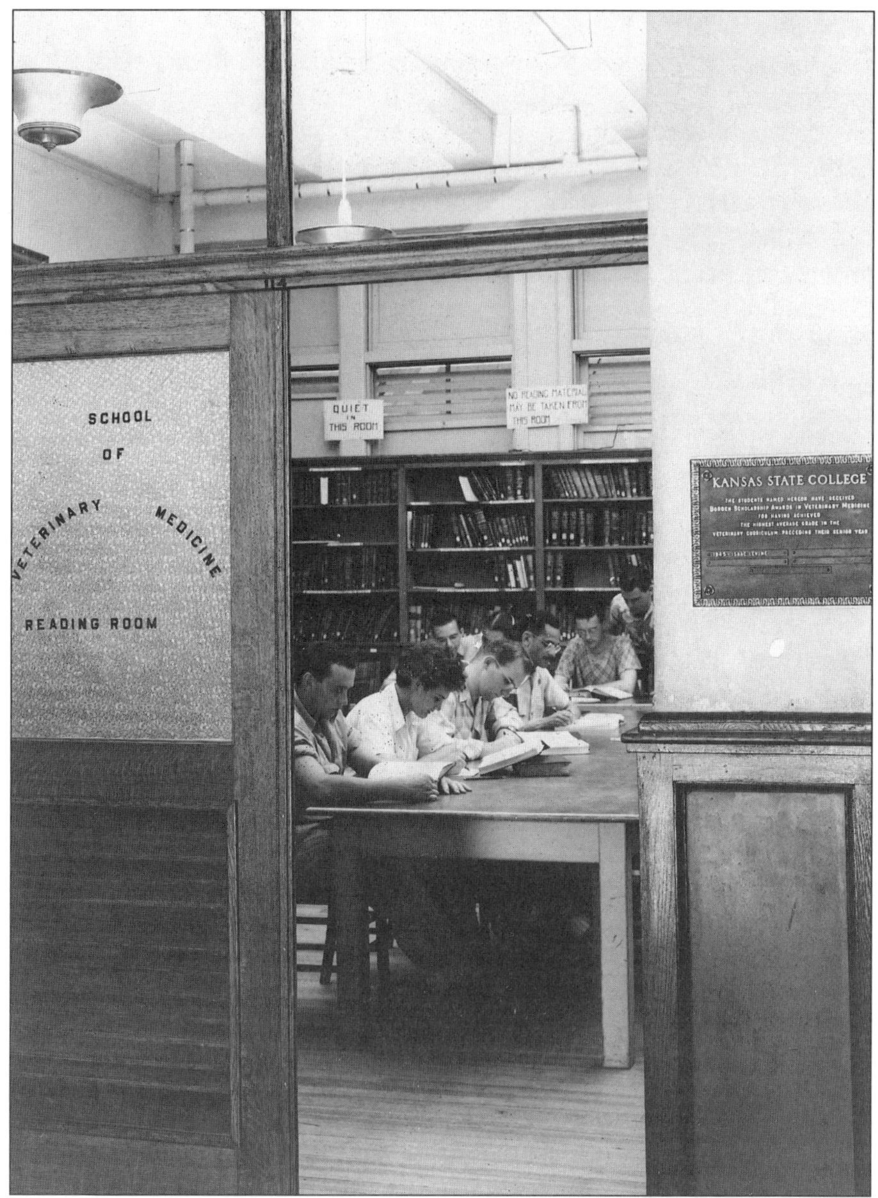

Phyllis with classmates in the Reading Room, circa 1946

her out in the group exclaiming, "Give her the bottle. Let her try." Not one to let the side down, Phyllis with all eyes focused on her, straddled the calf, backed it to a wall, stuck a finger in it's mouth gently sliding the nipple in beside it and before you knew it was sucking. Mr. Casement whooped out "By God, I knew it! The maternal instinct! It never fails." Phyllis felt quite sure that having had her first dairy calf at age four to take care of had something to do with it!

One summer, Phyllis found herself gathering and recording eggs at the poultry houses, where groups of hens were used in production experiments. She was one of three students taking a summer Poultry Anatomy class for graduate credit. One other student, a Dr. Mobiley, was from the brand new school of veterinary medicine at Tuskegee. Upon finishing their course Dr. Mobiley conferred to Phyllis that he wished he could have invited her to teach with him at Tuskegee when she had finished her veterinary degree at Kansas State. He added that he could not because at that time it was illegal to mix races on faculties in Alabama. This was quite something to Phyllis, who thought at times she was discriminated against for being a woman, but not because of her race!

Phyllis was a great observer of people and even though not always seeing their point of view, liked to see the good in them.

She enjoyed her professors and remembers many of them for different reasons. Dr. E. J. Frick, who liked to challenge students by saying outrageous things, was a surprisingly good judge of people. Phyllis

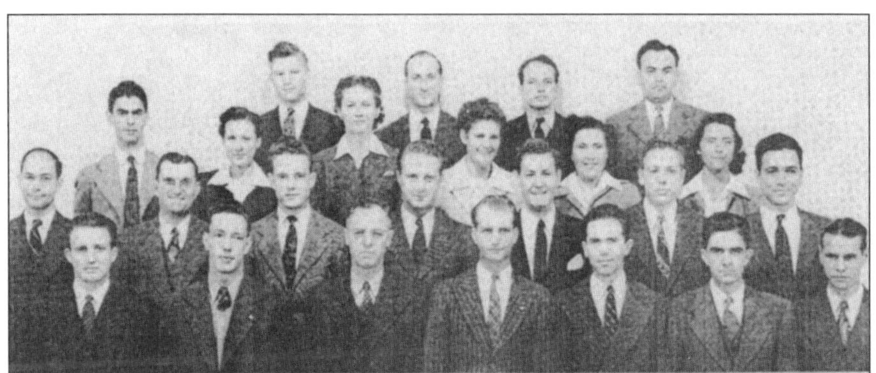

Phyllis her Freshman Year, with class members from both 1947 classes

remembers the day when Dr. Frick was lecturing the students about dealing with future bosses and employees. He explained, "Take George Cook (a student) for instance. You might have to push him to do something. On the other hand, take Miss Hickney. Don't ever try to push her, or she won't do anything. You have to convince her that she wants to do it."

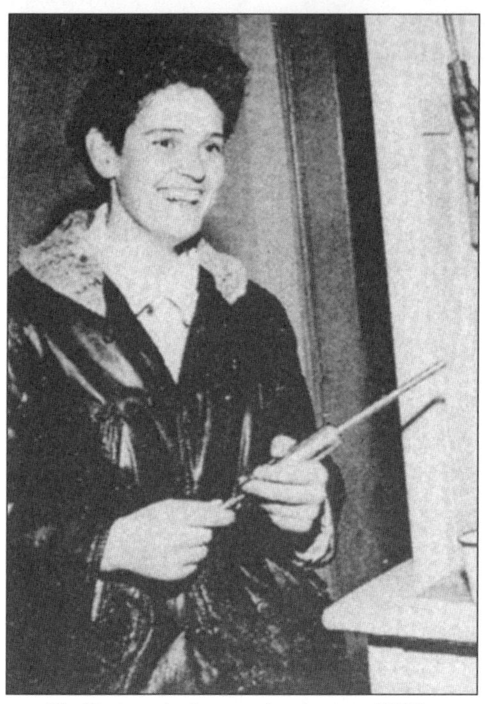

Phyllis in veterinary school, circa 1947

Phyllis remembers so much about her veterinary school days and the people who made it memorable. One such person was Dr. W. M. McLeod, a kind and thoughtful man. When Phyllis felt herself separated from some of her classmates it was to Dr. McLeod that she turned. One such time came when some of her classmates thought she should be beaten for walking across campus with a Negro man. It was a good feeling for Phyllis to have a member of faculty to turn to with concerns. Phyllis felt she was fortunate to have very few worries, but so fortunate to have a trusted mentor as Dr. McLeod.

Dr's Roderick, Moore, Cover and even old Dr. Burt were all remembered as gentlemen that Phyllis appreciated.

Phyllis had no time for socializing in a great way, especially if it involved dressing up. She remembers the one and only time she rose to the occasion whilst in veterinary school. Every year the Junior Association Veterinary Medical Association as it was then (SCAVMA as it is now) hosted a reception in honor of the seniors. Phyllis, who had recently disappointed the Dean by not showing up for her installation into Phi Kappa Phi, felt maybe she should make the effort. First of all there was of course the dress issue. This was kindly resolved by the kindness of her landlady Mrs. Fenton, providing Phyllis with a gown. Phyllis had lived with the Fenton's during her last year of veterinary school, in exchange for room and board she kept the bathroom neat, cleaned the house weekly and was responsible for keeping the family's pet fox terrier "Butch" bathed when needed.

Not wanting to show up in a beautiful gown without a date seemed dull, so Phyllis invited a junior student by the name of Johnny Aiken. Johnny, who's fiancé was back East, was quite comfortable in going to the reception with the most 'attractive tomboy' in veterinary school!

Phyllis had worked hard during her three years of veterinary school, involving herself with Student Government, and was a member of Gamma Sigma Delta and Phi Kappa Phi. On June 1, 1947, Dr. Phyllis Hickney, alongside her friend Mary Hammond and twenty-one men, accepted her veterinary degree.

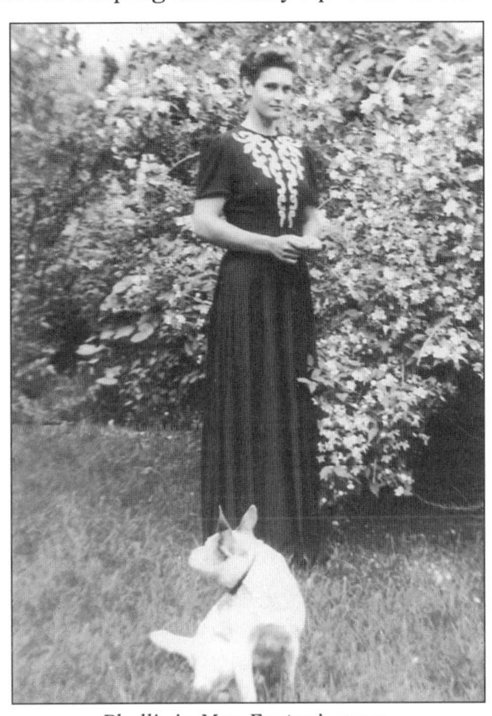

Phyllis in Mrs. Fenton's gown, with "Butch" looking on, May 1947

Phyllis accepted a position at Cornell, in Ithaca, New York, following her graduation. Here she worked at a veterinary experiment station of the United States Department of Agriculture. It was at Cornell that Phyllis authored and co-authored three papers. The October 1950 issue of Cornell Veterinarian, featured the paper Phyllis authored, entitled *Opsonic Indexes Of Cattle Following A Brucella Abortus Bacterin*.

It was at Cornell that she met Charles M. Larsen, a teaching fellow in Mathematics. On October 10, 1948, Phyllis and Charles were married at Myrtle Beach, South Carolina.

The following year, in 1949, they were blessed with the birth of a baby girl, Kristin Helga Larsen.

After three years at Cornell, Phyllis and her new husband moved to Palo Alto, in California, in 1950. Here Charles could further his studies at Stanford.

Phyllis spent the next few years having babies. Lawrence was born in 1951, and Ragnfrid (pronounced like Ronnie) born in 1953 and William, born in 1956.

Phyllis was kept busy as a volunteer or student during her children's school years, never far from animals. She worked part-time at the San Diego Zoological Gardens doing diagnostic work and autopsies for a couple of years.

Phyllis's son William remembered one fall day in 1973 when a hic-up in his social standing took place. For several weeks the head cheerleader had been giving William rides home after their high school football games. He decided to invite her in to meet the family prior to having her over for dinner in the future. He was crushed when he and the young lady stepped into the backyard patio to see a large dissected goose adorning the family's ping pong table. Phyllis, who was considered the neighborhood's veterinarian, took care of the many sick or injured animals. However, to arrive home with a future date to find your mother undergoing an impromptu autopsy did not look good. Phyllis was determined to find out the exact cause of death, rather than accept the simple "hit by car" explanation. Well, needless to say any romantic intentions suffered a severe blow when William's future girlfriend was reluctant to accept any dinner invitations. She insisted from here on out that William shop and prepare the food himself!

Phyllis's daughter Kristin remembers spending precious time with her mother at the San Diego Zoo. She remembered her mother caring for neighbor's animals and sharing her knowledge with many children, not just her own. Her mother was the 'nature counselor' at scout camps and a 4-H etymology advisor. Kristen was proud to have her mother pass on an insatiable curiosity about everything in life.

Daughter Ragnfrid, remembers being a girl scout and her mother being a wonderful leader, sharing her knowledge with so many young girls. Ragni is sure that there are many women veterinarians today because of her mother.

Ragni is sure that her mother's honorable ways go way back to possibly Native American inheritance. She is proud to have such a giving, caring mother.

During the years 1976–1977, Phyllis spent time with Mac on his sabbatical at Brown University and Cornell libraries. Phyllis searched for material on goats in health and disease. The ending result was a beginning bibliography on goats. Along with this Phyllis co-authored a paper on goats as research animals. She delivered the paper at a National Lab Animal Association meeting in 1979.

What Phyllis would not try. In 1981, she earned her MPVM from University of California, Davis. Her thesis was on the feral goats of San Clemente Island and their diseases. This led to a paper at the 4th International Conference on Goats at Tuscon, Arizona, in 1982.

As a young child, Phyllis had a love for China, and had always wanted to visit this wonderful place. Mac promised Phyllis that he would visit China with her Phyllis in turn, promised Mac she would learn to play bridge. Mac released Phyllis from her end of the bargain after a couple of tries. Mac though kept his end of the bargain.

Phyllis's dream to visit China came true in 1984 when she was to teach English at Beijing (Now Chinese National) Agricultural University. Mac was to follow later and taught mathematics for biologists.

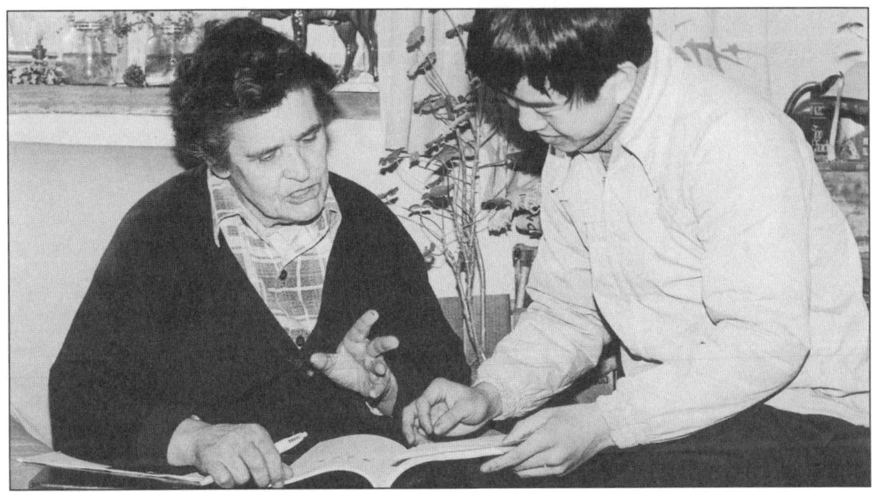

Phyllis with veterniary student Chen Xianhai,
at Beijing Agricultural University, circa 1986-1987

In 1987, Phyllis and Mac retired back to Ithaca, New York. Here they both could enjoy the colorful autumns and snowy winters they so missed.

Phyllis probably would say that she has not achieved so much in her life. Adding the years that both she and Mac devoted to the national office of the American Association of Small Ruminant Practitioners, and time serving as President of the American Veterinary History Society (1999--2000), and compiling a history book for the Association for Women Veterinarians published in 1997, I believe she has achieved much.

Putting aside all her career achievements and veterinary associations, I believe that Phyllis's greatest achievement is the knowledge she has passed on to so many people. We talk of modern day mentors, if there ever was a founder of these, it was Phyllis. Phyllis has a unique way of looking at life, respecting the differences we all have and always looking for the remarkable qualities we might share. As her daughter Kristen quite plainly said, "If my mother had not embraced the unusual, she might not have considered a career in veterinary medicine." After all, it was not a common choice for women at that time, and Phyllis definitely wasn't common!

To Hold Its Own
If I were pushed
to carve one thought on lasting stone,
I'd say,
 "I trust we come from stuff that's
 tough enough to hold its own."

–Written by Dr. Phyllis "Hickney" Larsen in 1965.

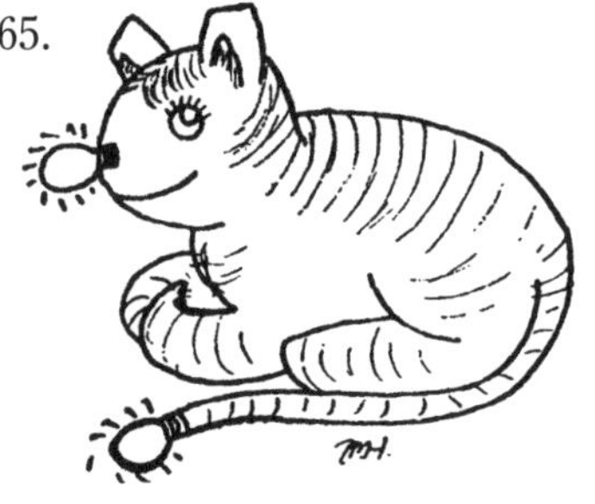

Phyllis Mae Hickney
Chronology

1923: 26 March, born Worcester, Massachusetts.

1940: Graduated from David Prouty High School, Spencer, Massachusetts

1944: Received AB (Zoology) from Vassar.
Admitted to the Professional Curriculum at Kansas State College, School of Veterinary Medicine.

1947: 1 June, Graduated from veterinary school at Kansas State College.

1948: 10 September, Married Charles M. Larsen, Myrtle Beach, South Carolina.

1949: 11 June, Birth of daughter Kristin Helga.

1950: Moved to Palo Alto, California.

1951: 22 May, Birth of son Lawrence Charles.

1953: 14 October, Birth of daughter Ragnfrid Jean.

1956: 3 March, Birth of son Wm. Davis McLoud.

92

1981 : Earned MPVM, from University of California, Davis.

1984-
1987 : Taught English to Veterinarians and others in China.

1987 : Retired and moved back to Ithaca, New York.

1996 : American Association of Small Ruminants, Veterinarian of the Year.

1999 : Served as President of the American Veterinary History Society.

2001 : Presented exhibit on Florence Kimball, DVM, RN (One of America's first female veterinarian), at AVMA convention.

2002 : Received the Judith Spurling Blue Ribbon Award from the Association of Women Veterinarians.

1999-
2000 : President of the American Veterinary Medical History Society.

Chapter 9

Margaret Patricia Denison
–1949 School of Veterinary Medicine
Kansas State College

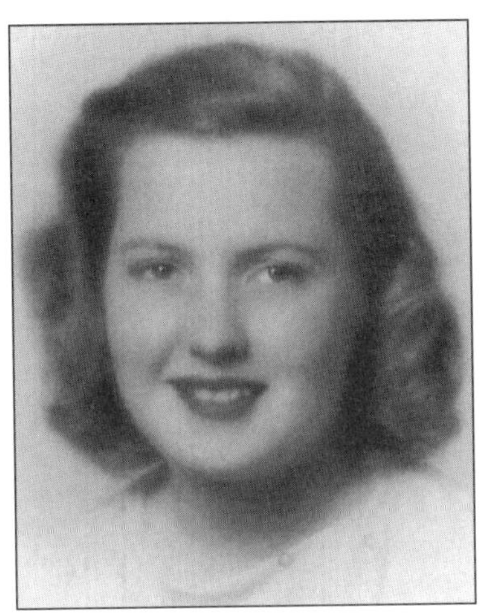

$\mathcal{M}$argaret Patricia Denison was born May 31, 1927, to William and Katherine (Troppman) Denison, at St. Johns Hospital in Chippewa Falls, Wisconsin. She was the only child born to this union, having two step-brothers, Robert and Jack and one step-sister, Wilma, from her father's previous marriage.

The mere fact that William "Doc" Denison was a veterinarian and owned horses probably had some influence on the 'spunky' petite "Patsy" (as she was nicknamed).

Doc Denison had graduated from veterinary school in Chicago in the early 1900's. He located to Bemidji, Minnesota where he practiced for many years at his Denison Veterinary Hospital.

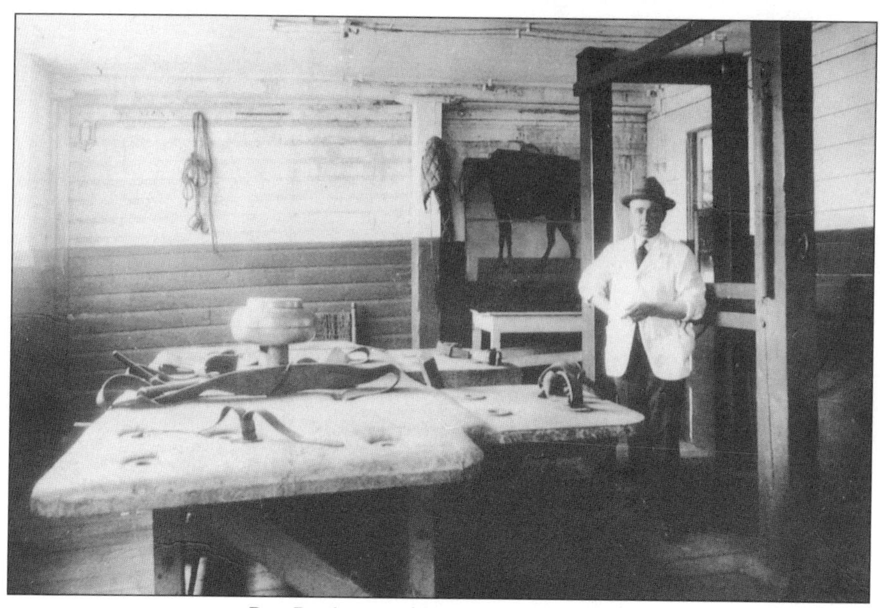

Doc Denison, at his veterinary hospital

Doc Denison had Patsy ride along with him on his farm and house calls. She became his first 'young assistant'. Not only did the young Patsy learn the practice of veterinary medicine, but the practice of selling vehicles, as her father also owned the Chevrolet and Buick agency in Bemidji, Minnesota.

Patsy spent her elementary years growing up with her parents, grandparents and other relatives in Bemidji, Minnesota. There was nothing more fun for Patsy than to ride along with her father in the historically charming and beautiful city. She would attend the local schools and obtained good grades.

It was the great passion for horses that Patsy acquired from her father. Having two associates in his practice (Basil S. Swink, and Josiah A. Given), gave Doc the time to spend with Patsy and their horses.

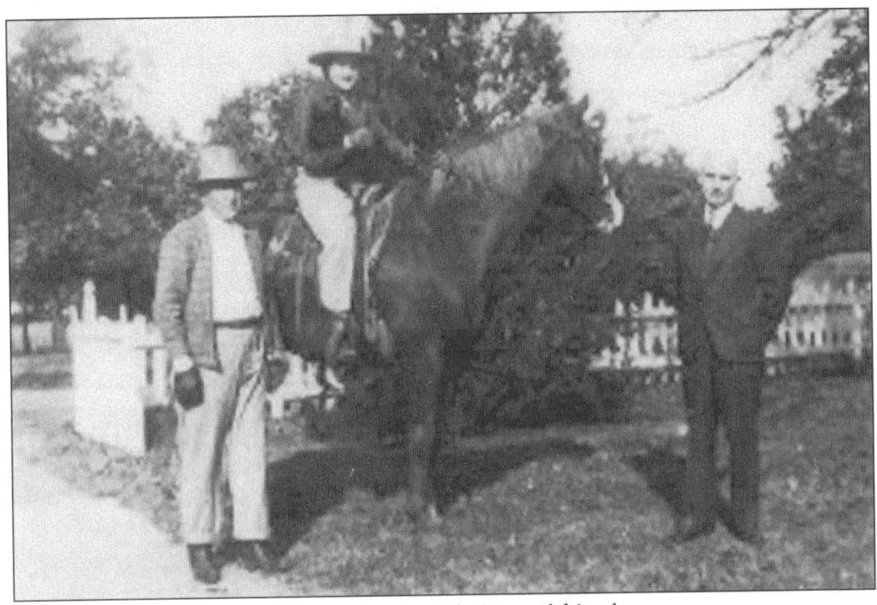

Patsy on horse, with Doc and friend

Patsy loved all species of animals, but her favorite was the horse. One of her favorite pastimes was to barrel race. She won several ribbons racing her Pinto horse "Popcorn". Patsy was never more proud than when she rode Popcorn in parades and at the rodeos.

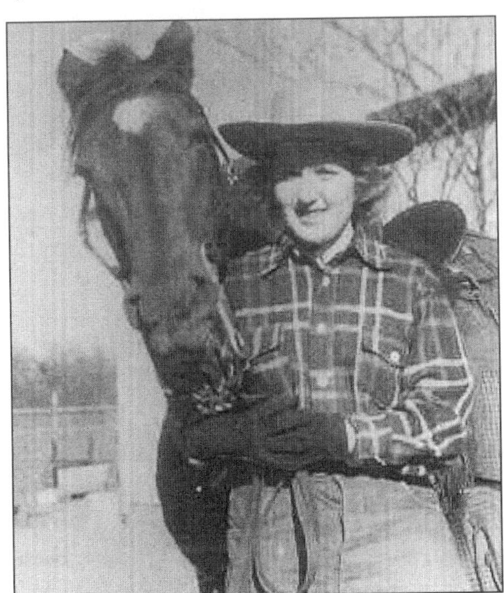

Patsy with one of her favorite horses

When Patsy wasn't with her father and the horses, she could be found downtown at Grandpa Troppmans store. The store sold dry goods, rubber boots, winter underwear and many irregular items. It was most definitely a haven for a young child like Patsy! Her mother Katherine kept books for her father at the store.

Painting was another pastime of Patsy's. She enjoyed painting mostly animals and people.

It was sometime before Patsy's junior year in high school that Doc retired from his veterinary practice. The family re-located to Oklahoma City, Oklahoma, in 1942.

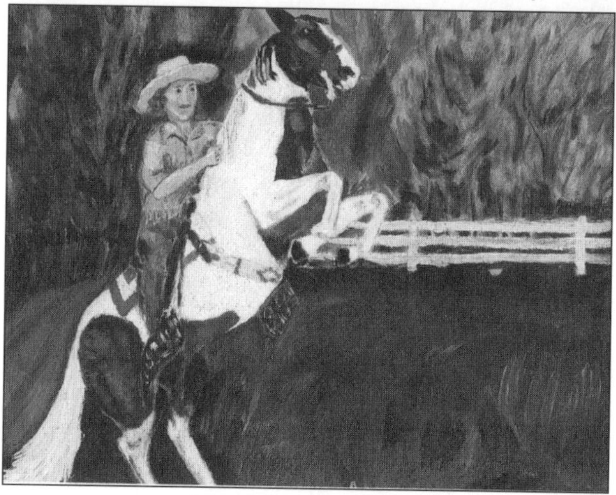
One of Patsy's paintings

Re-locating meant that Patsy would finish her last two years of high school at Central High School, in Oklahoma City. She graduated with the class of 1944.

Patsy knew that she wanted to work with animals, especially with horses. It was with the influence and support of her father, Doc Denison, that she would be admitted to the Pre-veterinary curriculum at Kansas State College, School of Veterinary Medicine, in 1944. One year later in 1945 she was admitted to the Professional Curriculum.

Patsy worked and enjoyed her time in veterinary school. She was be remembered by classmates, Dr's Kay, Fishburn, Kennedy, and Woolsey, as a congenial class member. Patsy was described as being a nice girl, competent and an extremely good sport!

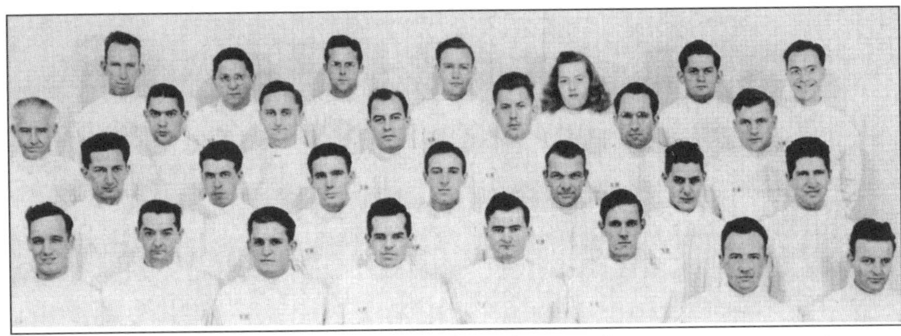

Patsy with some of her class members

The class of 1949 was made up of men who had been rejected from military service, men who had early separation from the military, and one female. Patsy and other class members may well have not been admitted to Kansas State had it not been for WW II. Even though the war was concluding, there were few Kansas boys to fill the classes, thus opening a door for Patsy and men from out-of-state. Patsy was thankful for this and worked hard to obtain her veterinary degree.

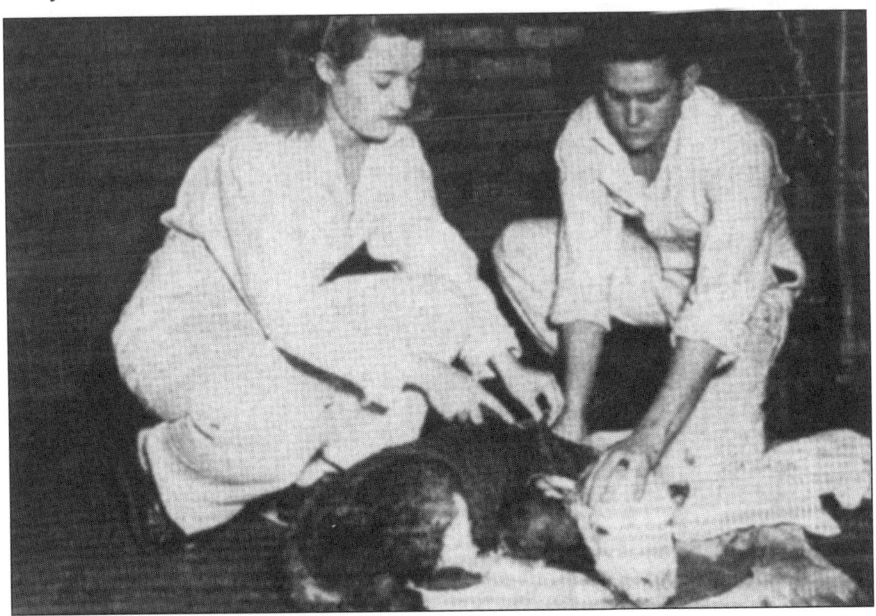

Patsy treating a calf in veterinary school

Dr. Margaret Patricia Denison graduated with fifty-nine men on the 29 May, 1949.

This was a proud time for Patsy's parents, having their daughter follow in her father's footsteps. Doc Denison built a veterinary hospital in Scottsville, Virginia for Patsy to practice out off. It was near to the farm that Doc owned and Patsy was able to take care of their horses.

It was a busy few years for Patsy, working and eventually becoming a mother to a daughter, Louise, born July 23, 1954. Being a single mother and working offered its challenges, but Patsy muddled through as best she could.

Sadly Patsy developed health problems that prevented her from practicing, and retired permanently from practice in about 1957.

It was on January 29, the following year that Patsy lost her father Doc W. K. Denison to a heart attack.

Even though Patsy is unable to say herself, her daughter Louise will tell you that, for as proud that her mother is of her two grandchildren and three great-grandchildren, she is every bit as proud to have graduated from Kansas State College, School of Veterinary Medicine.

Margaret Patricia Denison
Chronology

1927: May 31, Margaret Patricia Denison was born in St. John's Hospital, Chippewa Falls, Wisconsin, to William Denison and Catherine (Troppman) Denison.

1942: Parents moved to Oklahoma City, Oklahoma

1944: Graduated from Central High School, Oklahoma City, Oklahoma.

1944: Admitted to the Pre-veterinary Curriculum at Kansas State College, School of Veterinary Medicine.

1945: September 25, admitted to the Professional Curriculum at Kansas State College, School of Veterinary Medicine.

1949: May 29, graduated alongside 59 men from the School of Veterinary Medicine, Kansas State College.

Opened veterinary hospital in Scottsville, VA

1954: July 23, daughter Louise born.

1957: Retired from veterinary practice due to health problems.

1958: Patsy's father W. K. "Doc" Denison passed away.

Chapter 10

Dorothy Claire "Dixon" Fockele
–1951 School of Veterinary Medicine
Kansas State College

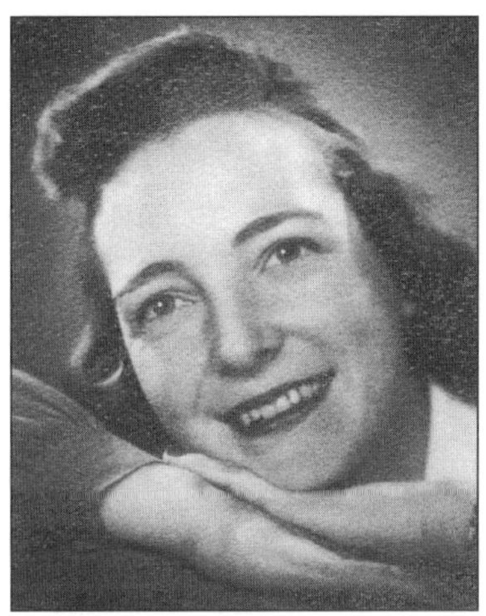

Dorothy Claire Dixon was the fourth child born to Nicholas John Dixon and Margaret "Hubbard" Dixon, on October 7, 1918 in Detroit, Michigan.

Nicholas worked as a court clerk, while Margaret worked as a seamstress and homemaker.

"Dottie," as Dorothy was nicknamed, along with her older sisters Lee and Esther, and brother Robert attended the public schools in Detroit.

As a young child Dottie was sickly, and having breathing problems, was sent to live with her mother's brother and his family on their farm in New Baltimore, Michigan. The farm was considered to be a healthier environment than the city for the small child.

Even though she skipped third grade, Dottie thrived on the farm. She loved the daily routine of learning to milk and care for the sheep, poultry, cats and dogs. Learning to ride the great draft horses was a tonic in itself. Once her health improved she returned to her schooling in Detroit.

Whenever she could Dottie returned to spend time at the farm. She loved the animals, especially the horses.

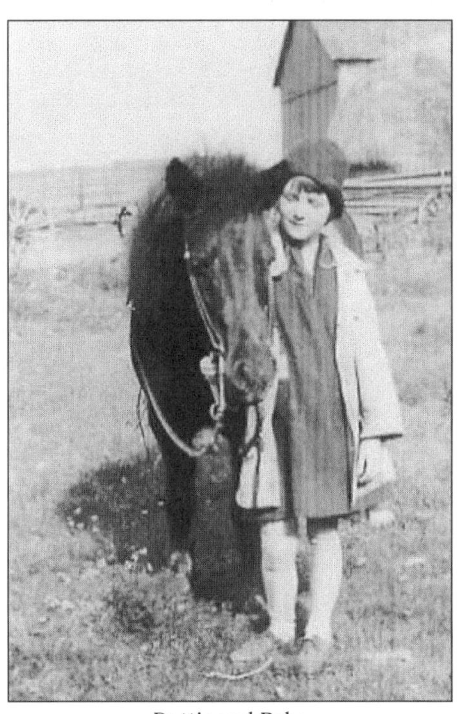

Dottie and Babe

Kiddies Mourn Loss Of Pony That Was Pet

Dorothy Dixon and her coterie of little friends in New Baltimore don't seem to find the sun shining quite as brightly now as it did the first of the week. Something is lacking when they gather on the Dixon lawn for a rollicking time that fails to prove so hilarious.

Investigation reveals that they have a right to feel lonesome and blue.

Dorothy Dixon's pet pony "Babe" died Tuesday and the children lost a real friend.

Dottie was a bright, smart and a very likeable girl, having many good friends. Her parents had raised her well, making sure she had a good education, and a family that loved her.

In her senior year in high school Dottie wrote a poem that clearly showed that her Catholic upbringing had made her a thankful and *'contented'* young woman.

It was in June, 1936 that John and Margaret were proud to see their daughter Dottie graduate Summa cum Laude, from Saint Leo High School, in Detroit. Dottie was also proud to accept a scholarship to Mount St. Joseph College, Cincinnati in Ohio.

It was while attending Mount St. Joseph College that Dorothy's name appeared in the Detroit News. Sometime in January of 1937, Dorothy along with two hundred other girls, watched anxiously as the Ohio River swelled its banks, flooding the valley surrounding it. The College, sitting high on a hill, was safe from flood waters but was evacuated because of dangers of pestilence and disease. The newspaper account described the devastation to the homes and businesses. Dorothy recounted the efforts of the Red Cross and how she and the girls assisted them, making bandages from blankets. The college girls also cared for more than eighty orphans who were rescued from a Cincinnati orphanage.

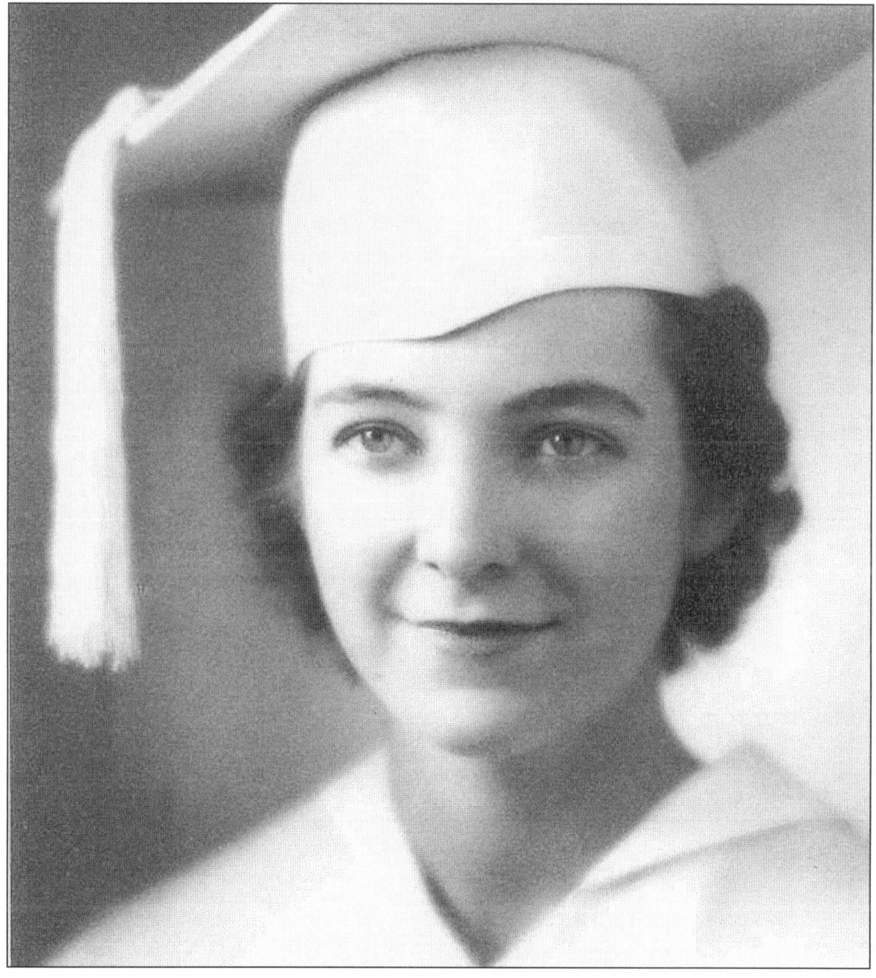

Dottie in 1936, St. Leo's High School

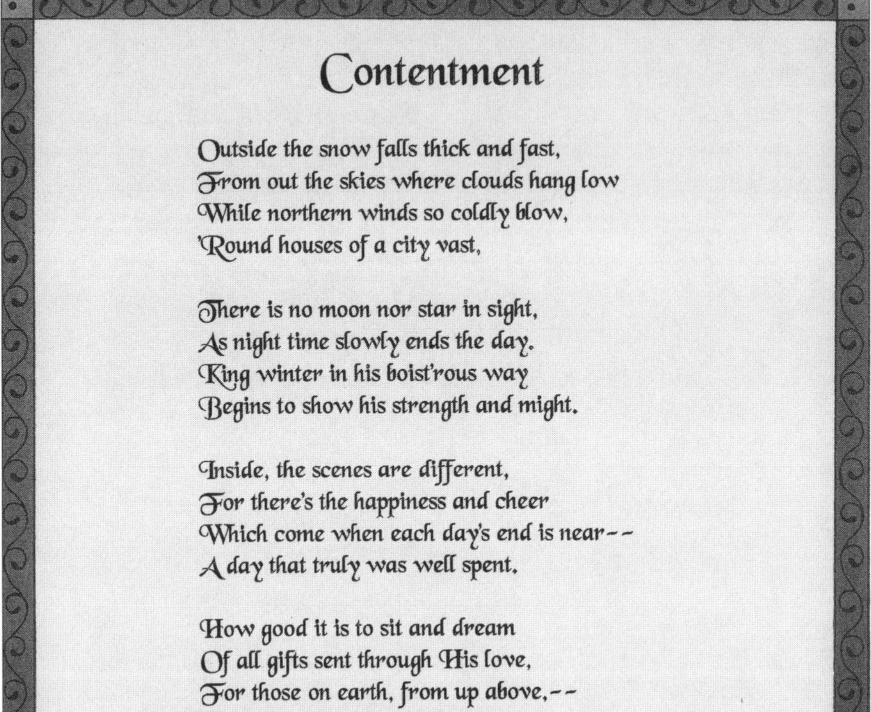

Dottie enjoyed Mount St. Joseph College, though after a year she transferred to Michigan State. It was here that she became a member of the Alpha Phi Sorority (an international network of sisters, based on encouragement, understanding and a growth). Dottie excelled here in horsemanship, even placing second in the college horse show. She was proud of her favorite mount, a horse called 'Wonderful Boy,' a striking chestnut with a white stripe down his nose.

Dottie was an attractive young woman, with tomboy characteristics. She enjoyed, like most young people did in the late thirties, the sounds of

Glenn Miller and Benny Goodman. In her sophomore year Dottie was honored to be prom leader, her date for the evening was Ted Mackrell, a gentleman from New York.

Dottie's summers were spent at Camp Cavell, a YWCA camp on Lake Huron in Michigan. She had started as a camper back in high school and was now Chief Instructor. She was happy to be paid the sum of seventy-five dollars for two months work as Senior Riding Counselor.

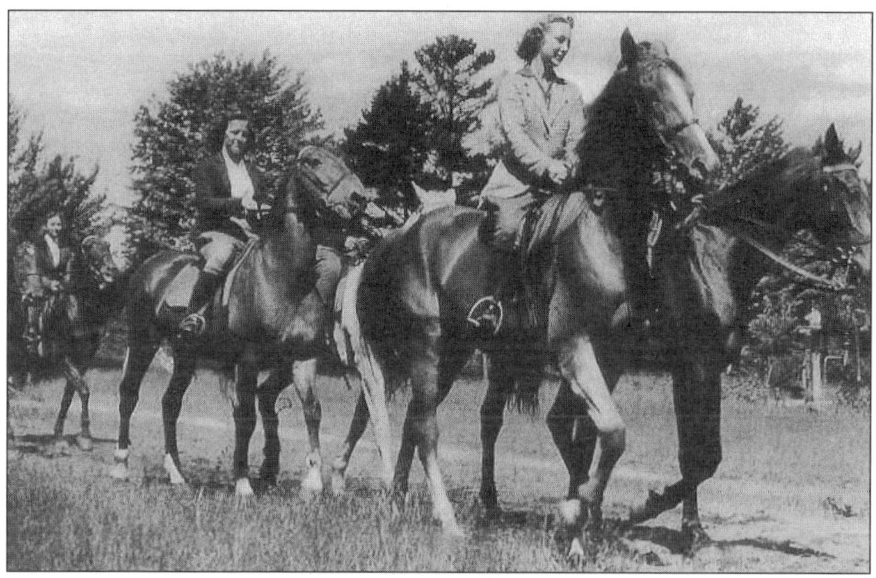

Dottie at Camp Cavil

Dottie graduated from Michigan State with a degree in Animal Science, on June 10, 1940. From here she found secretarial work, something she really did not enjoy. In about 1942 Dottie moved to Nebraska where she lived with her sister Lee and her husband.

With World War Two underway, many jobs opened for the women. Dottie was proud to do her part and worked as a 'Rosie the Riveter' (women worked on assembly lines riveting airplane parts, fastening them together with metal pins) for a year and a half at The Glenn L. Martin – Nebraska Company, in Omaha, Nebraska. She was honored to be presented with a certificate as testament of her loyal and faithful service to war work.

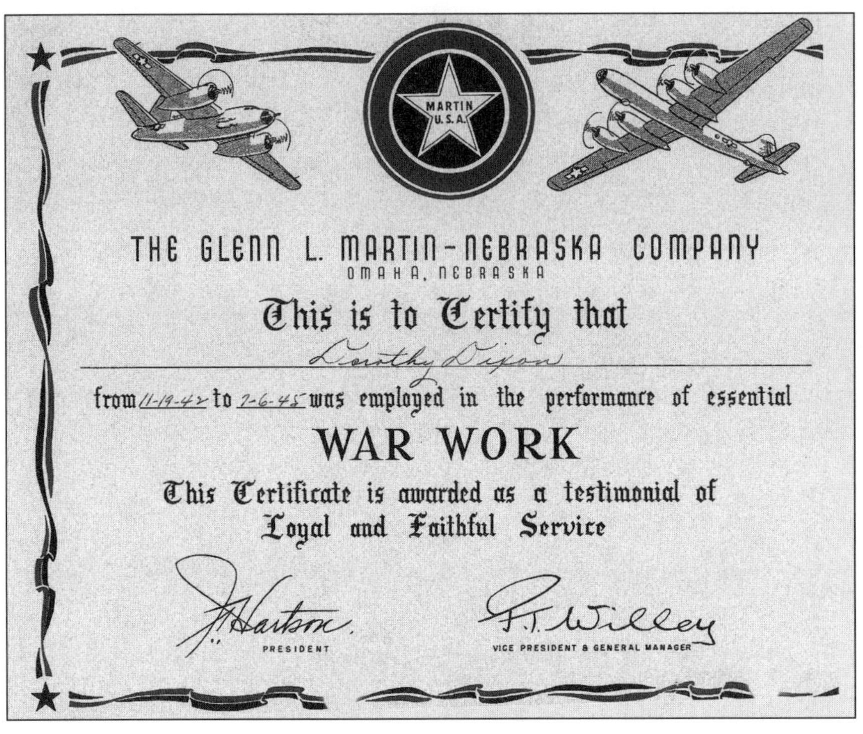

Dottie was a firm believer in women being able to choose their course in life, their given abilities and talents should not be denied because of their gender or race! For a young woman, raised in the 1920's and 1930's, this was quite an attitude!

What Dottie would not try! It was during the war, while living in Nebraska that she became familiar with the 'bush league' racetracks. She worked as a hot walker (walking the horses after exercise to cool them down) and exercise girl. Being only four foot and eleven inches, Dottie was the perfect rider to exercise the horses. Having the men away at war meant that she was in demand.

It was at the tracks that Dottie was inspired to want to become a veterinarian. She did not like to see the horses abused. The atrocities of trainers drugging and injecting sick horses to get them through races disgusted her. Appalled at the abuse of the animals, Dottie applied to veterinary school at Kansas State College. She was determined to make a difference in the life of animals, especially horses.

Dottie applied to Kansas State College, as it had the last remaining co-ed mounted cavalry unit. This meant that she could ride the officer's horses on a regular basis whilst in school.

She was happy to be accepted to the professional curriculum on September 25, 1945.

Dottie arrived in Manhattan, Kansas with a suitcase and a horse named Pharalea that she had purchased from a track back in Nebraska.

Dottie enjoyed her classes and worked hard. She enjoyed participating in the educational and social events of the Student Chapter of the American Veterinary Medical Association.

Like some of the earlier women, Dottie had to contend with disparaging remarks from some of the men. They were of the opinion that such a slight female was better suited in a different profession. Dottie, however, was of the opinion that she was there to learn about the diseased or injured animal, not to show how well she could grapple it to the ground. One professor agreed with her, making sure the male counterpart realized that Dottie was doing the right thing, "observing and examining before making a wrong move!"

While in veterinary school, Dottie met a veterinary student by the name of William Rex Fockele. Bill or 'Doc' as he was later called, was a returning war veteran, having served for four years in the marines. Doc was a native of Ottawa, Kansas.

Doc fell in love with Dottie and of course Pharalea! Doc and Dottie were united in marriage September 25, 1945, in the Rectory at the church of the Seven Dolors, Manhattan, Kansas.

Doc and Dottie lived for a year or so in a silver trailer home at Ninth and Colorado in Manhattan. They enjoyed the company of a new Dalmatian puppy, Lucky and Pharalea who was housed in a chicken coop next to their trailer.

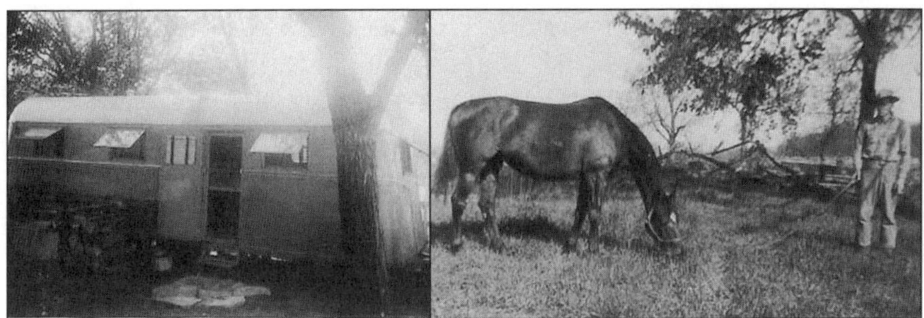

At home in Manhattan

They were blessed with a new addition to their family October 31, 1947, this time not an animal, but a baby boy Bill.

Dottie was concerned that she may have to drop out of veterinary school, but was encouraged by Doc and his mother not to. (Having a mother-in-law near-by was a blessing)!

After Doc's graduation in May of 1949, they moved to Salina, Kansas, where Doc opened a practice. Later that same year they were blessed again with a second son Nick, born December 26.

Dottie had worked hard in school, and attained outstanding grades. She missed graduation with her class of 1949 by having her babies, but proudly accepted her veterinary degree January 26, 1951, after making up her missed classes. She was the only veterinary student to accept a degree at this mid-term commencement.

The Dr.'s Fockele enjoyed working together for awhile in Salina, and raising their two sons.

Doc shared Dottie's passion for horses and was excited to see an ad in the Bloodhorse magazine for an equine practioner at the prestigious Mereworth Farm in Kentucky. He was delighted when he applied and was hired.

Dottie, Doc and the boys moved in late spring 1951 to Lexington, Kentucky. Within a few months of settling in baby girl Suzy arrived, on August 10.

Doc stayed busy and consulted with Dottie on his many cases, his being the final decision as he was the hired veterinarian.

Dottie stayed busy with her children, devoting herself to being a housewife. Her days were only to become busier! On August 27, 1952 baby son Bob was born, followed October 20, 1953 by baby boy Dan, followed by baby girl

Mary born September 26, 1955. Two years later, baby girl Jane was born on June 15, 1958. A few years later in June of 1961, little baby Helen was born. Sadly due to a difficult birth, she only lived for a few days.

Dottie's Catholic upbringing influenced her to focus on her family first and her passion for horses and veterinary medicine second.

Dr. Dottie enjoyed spending any time she could with the horses. She was especially honored one year when a colt by the famous horse Native Dancer had ran into a fence, causing a nasty facial injury. Being a well bred colt and having potential for breeding purposes, his owners wished to save him. Doc had contacted a couple of his and Dottie's former professors at Kansas State, and was delighted when they joined him to perform surgery to save the colt. Dottie was to assist too.

Doc and Dottie worked side by side, daughter Suzy remembers. It was delicate surgery requiring good technique and expertise. Dottie was in her element. Young Suzy was proud to be allowed to stay home and watch her parents complete the necessary surgery.

If Dottie could not be practicing, she kept up on what was going on in the veterinary world by reading. She loved to read, reading was one of her favorite hobbies, besides riding. Daughter Suzy remembers her mother reading magazines such as The Smithsonian and National Geographic cover to cover.

Dottie loved her time with her children and as they grew and one by one left home, she and Doc turned to bird watching as a hobby.

In 1969 Dottie was diagnosed with breast cancer; it was a battle she was to fight for the next twenty - three years. Dottie passed away July 12, 1992 in Kentucky.

The hard working little Dottie, who completed her veterinary degree when women were not so easily accepted to the profession, rose to the challenge and stayed focused on her chosen career. If Dottie could, she would probably tell you that the happiest days of her life were spent with Doc at Kansas State!

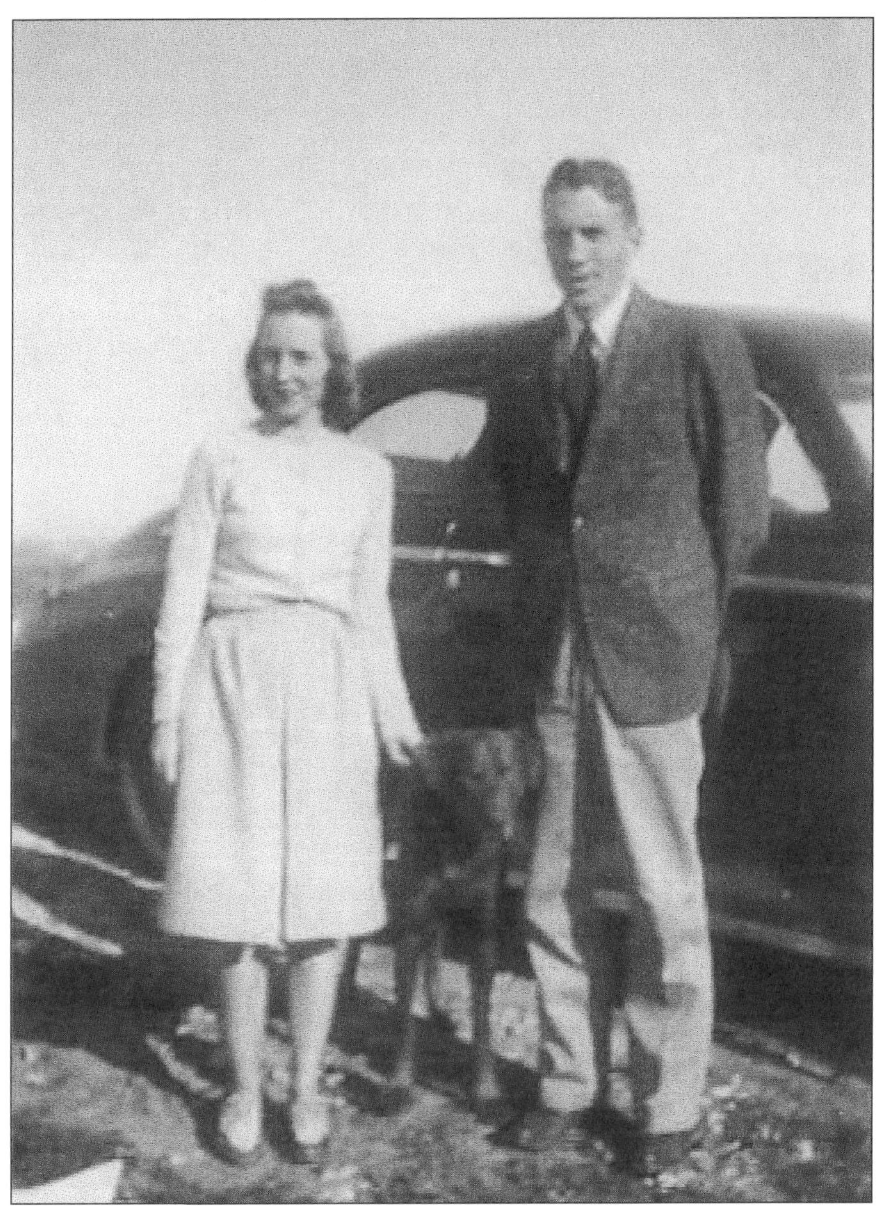

Dottie and William

Dorothy Claire "Dixon" Fockele
Chronology

1918: 7 October, 1918 born in Detroit, Michigan.

1936: 14 June, graduated from St Leo High School, in Michigan.
Attended Mount St. Joseph College, in Michigan.

1940: 10 June, graduated from Michigan State, with degree in Animal Science.

1941: Summer, Senior Riding Counselor, Camp Cavell, Michigan

1942–1945: 19 November through 7 June, employed at Glenn L. Martin Company in Nebraska, as a 'Rosy the Riveter.'

1945: 25 September, admitted to professional curriculum, Kansas State College, School of Veterinary Medicine.

1946: 23 November, married William Rex Fockele, Manhattan, Kansas.

1947: 31 October, son Bill born in Kansas.

1949: 20 May, husband William, graduated from KSCSVM.
26 December, son Nick born in Kansas.

1951 : 1 January, graduated from veterinary school.
10 August, daughter Suzy born in Kentucky.
Worked with Doc in their practice, in Salina, Kansas.
Moved with Doc to Mereworth Farm, Kentucky.

1952 : 27 August, son Bob born in Kentucky.

1953 : 20 October, son Dan born in Kentucky.

1955 : 26 September, daughter Mary born in Kentucky.

1958 : 15 June, daughter Jane born in Kentucky.

1961 : June, baby Helen born. Died within a few days of birth.

1962 : 12 July, passed away in Kentucky, following a long battle with
breast cancer.

Chapter 11

Joanne Gertrude Gross
–1953 School of Veterinary Medicine
Kansas State College

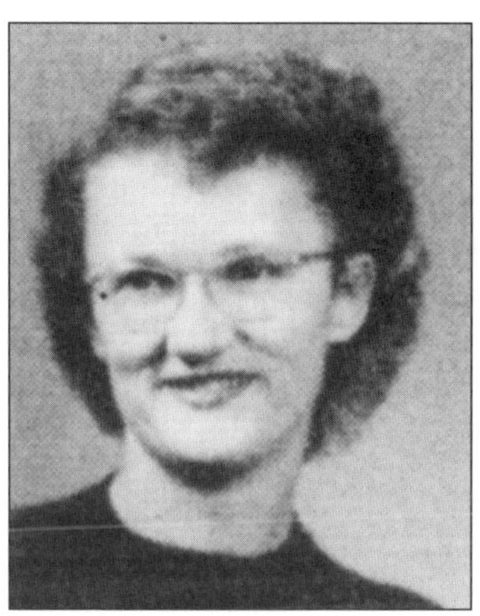

*J*oanne Gertrude Gross was born on November 21, 1928, to proud parents Norman J. Gross and Eva Mary "Cleveland" Gross, in Russell, Kansas.

Joanne was raised on the family farm alongside her brothers Joseph, Glenn, Dean, and William, and her sisters Virginia and Betty. In 1929, one more brother, Robert, arrived to complete the Gross family.

It was a good time on the farm, having an array of animals such as Black Angus cows, dairy cows, horses, pigs, sheep, chickens and ducks to take care of. Joanne also remembers the odd rattlesnake or two! Joanne's love for animals was apparent from a very young age. If she was not hanging on the neck of 'Nifty,' her favorite collie dog, she was out being cowgirl on her horse 'Dan'.

The family grew most of its own food. Some of the eggs and cream were taken into Russell and sold to Loren Dole, Bob Dole's father, who ran a produce store there.

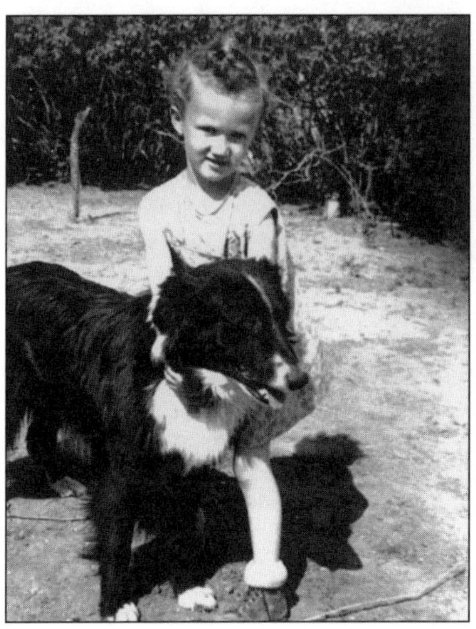

Joanne and Nifty, circa 1930's

Joanne attended the rural school house, which she remembers riding on horseback to each day, come rain or shine. She spent her teenage years attending Russell High School. Joanne and her siblings stayed with their grandmother in town during the week and returned home on the weekends. The school was a few blocks from their grandmother's, which made it easy for them to walk to.

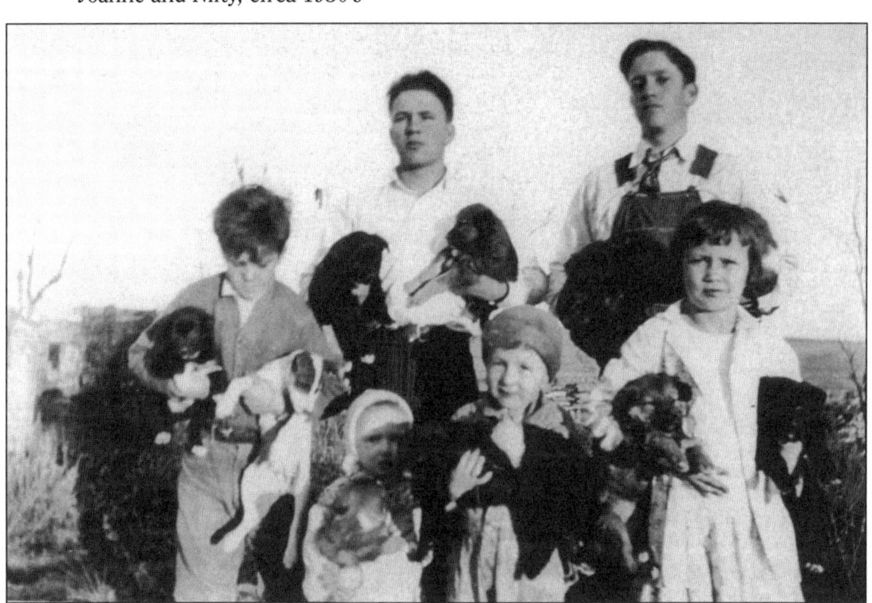

Joanne with siblings and puppies, circa 1929

The health of the Gross family animals was taken care of by Dr. H.D. O'Brien (graduate of Kansas City Veterinary College). The family enjoyed Dr. O'Brien, and later attributed his caring manner as inspiration for several of the Gross children who were making veterinary medicine their career of choice.

Education was an important factor in the Gross household. Joanne's father made sure that books were always available for the children to read. He was also on the school board of the one room schoolhouse she attended. He made sure the schoolchildren had a properly qualified teacher and the school had an adequate library.

In 1946, Joanne enrolled in the pre-veterinary curriculum at Kansas State College. Joanne's Grandmother Della Gross, a savvy business lady, had offered the Gross children five-thousand dollars each to either educate themselves or to spend as they saw fit. Joanne was happy to use her money for her education.

In Joanne's freshmen year she received Phi Kappa Phi recognition for good grades, she was in the upper ten percent of her class.

After completing two years of pre-vet Joanne was anxious to apply and follow in her brothers Glenn, Dean and

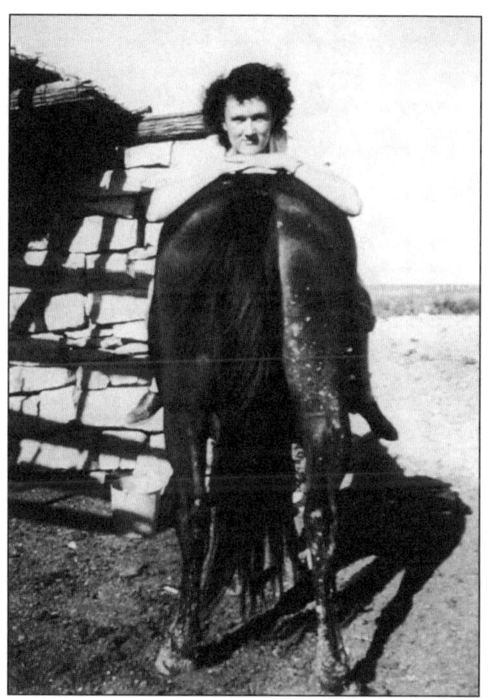

Ann a senior in high school

Williams's footsteps to become a veterinarian.

Joanne was disappointed to have her application to veterinary school turned down. Even though she had the required grades, she was told that preference was given to veterans! This accepted, she decided to go to school for one more year and apply again. In January 1949, alongside one other female Annie "Klena" Hurlburt, Joanne was admitted to veterinary school. She was happy to be accepted, but later as a Junior was sad to find out from one of her professors that she should have been accepted the first time she applied to veterinary school. The examining board had used the veterans as an excuse. In reality, they did not want females; they felt that women were taking jobs away from men! Joanne thought this was a load of B.S.! That's 'bad settlings,' according to Joanne's mother!

Joanne enjoyed her time in school and thought a lot of Dr's McLeod, Oberst, Frank and Mosier. She liked most of her classmates, but found some to be not so congenial.

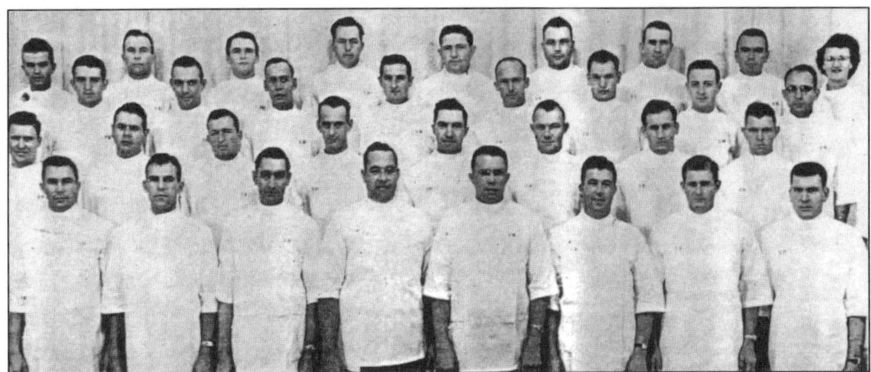

Joanne a Senior, with class members.

Joanne was a member of the Kansas State Chapter of the American Veterinary Medical Society.

She remembers her first year in veterinary school costing her slightly under seven hundred dollars, this included tuition, books, room and board .... everything. There was not much change left over for any extras.

A memorable incident happened after hours one day when Dr. Hay asked for a student to ride along with him on a large animal call. Joanne, knowing that she would miss supper at the dorm if she was not back in time, offered to go. On returning later, Dr. Hay found out that Joanne had missed supper and took her out to eat at Cohen's in Junction City. It was nice to be treated as a lady should be!

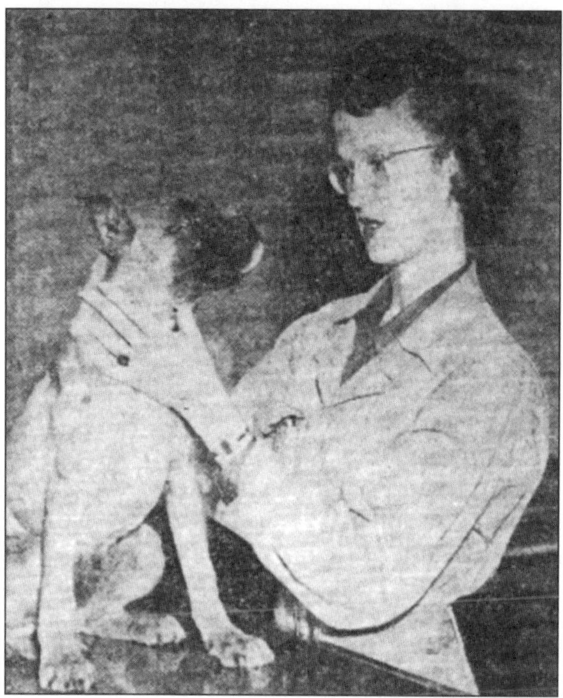

Dr. Joanne Gross (almost) April, 1953

Dr. Joanne Gross was happy to accept her veterinary degree on May 24, 1953, alongside sixty-five men. She was in the first group of students to graduate from the so called six year curriculum. Two years pre-veterinary and four years in the professional curriculum.

After graduation, Joanne joined her brothers Glenn, Dean and William in practice in Jacksonville, Illinois. Joanne, like her brothers, felt that there were better opportunities in Illinois than there were back home in Kansas. (Sadly, after the dustbowl and depression Kansas was dried up and offered little opportunity).

In 1952, her brother Robert graduated from veterinary school at Kansas State and set up a mixed practice in Virginia, Illinois. In 1966, Joanne persuaded him to join her in practice in Jacksonville.

On June 30, 1956 Joanne married William O. Deichmann, the marriage would last for twenty years before being dissolved.

Joanne was kept busy in the practice, working seven days a week for many years, eventually taking a Thursday afternoon off, and then all day. Her days working were spent doing small animal work and kennel work. She remembers inheriting all the chicken work in the practice, vaccinating and caponizing etc. Her hands being small, she was a dandy with obstetrical work in sheep and sows.

Each of the Gross veterinarians had an area of interest and skill, Joanne's was as a surgeon. In a newspaper article about the Gross's in 1997, Dean Gross mentioned that he and his brothers wanted 'Anne,' as they called her, along for caesareans because she was so neat and fast. In the same article, her brother Robert remembered the time he called Joanne to help with a heifer trying to calf. He needed her to assist with a caesarean. By the time Anne arrived, the owner of the heifer had called his friends and the rafters in the old barn that they were working in were full of workers! Joanne wished she could have charged for admission, feeling they would have made more on that than they did on the surgery!

It did not take Joanne long to realize that people were a big part of everything she did as a veterinarian. She remembers shortly after she started work in Jacksonville, a well dressed, polite gentleman came to her wanting to have his new Weimaraner puppy vaccinated and checked over for parasites etc. On leaving Joanne's office the gentleman inquired if he should pay now or wait until the puppy had finished his series of vaccinations. Joanne replied, "Now."

Joanne's office man asked her if she knew who the gentleman was? Her reply was "No." He explained that the gentleman was the president of Elliot State Bank and he probably would prefer to be billed monthly. From then on Joanne worked on his dog and told him that it was ok for him to make monthly payments. A few years later she was to ask this same gentleman at the Elliot State bank for a loan. She realized that for collateral she had little to offer. She was moving her clinic's location with one of her brothers, and her share was a dab over fifteen thousand dollars. The gentleman came and looked at the building and loaned Joanne the money. It was not until the gentleman's death that Joanne found out from his wife that he had loaned the money from his pocket. He knew with no collateral that the bank could not loan Joanne the money. The reason he loaned the money, his wife said, was because he liked the way Joanne ran her practice!

Joanne was made very happy on October 22, 1981 when she married Robert Pfeffer.

After her wedding Joanne continued to enjoy her patients and their owners until her retirement in 1985.

Today, you might find Joanne puttering in her garden with her fox terrier Penny. I am told she has a passion for growing many varieties of Iris, or 'Kansas Orchids' as her mother liked to call them.

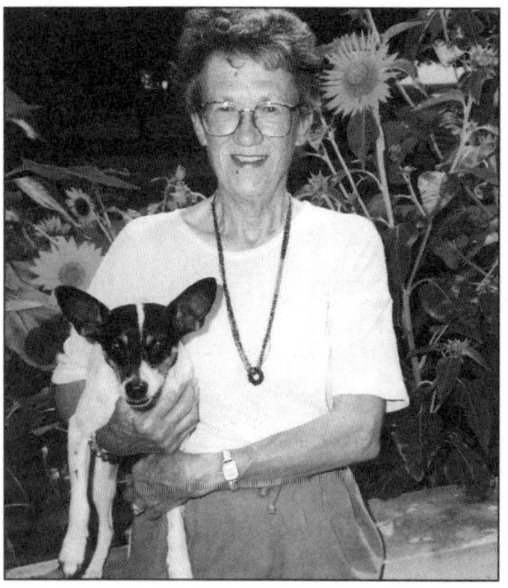
Dr. Joanne "Gross" Pfeffer, Penny
and Kansas Sunflowers

Dr. Robert Ulsh Gross, Joanne's youngest brother who is still in practice today wrote *A Veterinarians Limerick Book* in 1979. In this neat little book he dedicated this limerick to Joanne.

PARTNERS
My partner's the best that there be,
Although we don't always agree.
We do some quibbling,
She is my sibling.
A lady vet is she.

There is no doubt that Joanne left her mark on the veterinary profession. Her determination to become a veterinarian was apparent from the beginning; she never gave up even when turned down!

THE LADY IS A VETERINARIAN

Joanne Gertrude Gross
Chronology

1928 : 21 November, born in Russell, Kansas.

1939 : Brother Glenn G. Gross graduates D.V.M. from KSCSVM.

1944 : Brother Dean R. Gross graduates D.V.M. from KSCSVM.

1946 : May, graduated from Russell High School, Russell, Kansas.
September, enrolled at Kansas State College in Arts and Science.

1949 : 31 January, admitted to veterinary school, Kansas State College.

1950 : Brother William C. Gross graduates D.V.M. from KSCSVM.

1953 : 24 May, graduated Doctor of Veterinary Medicine. First group to graduate from six-year curriculum.
Joined brothers in practice in Jacksonville, Illinois.

1954 : Brother Robert U. Gross graduates D.V.M. from KSCSVM.

1956 : 30 June, Married to William O. Deichmann. Marriage dissolved after about 20 years.

1966 : 26 May, Joanne's father Norman Gross, passed away.

1970: 4 November, Joanne's mother Eva Gross, passed away.

1981: 22 October, married Robert Pfeffer.
(Robert passed away 16 December, 1999.)

1985: Retired from active practice.

Chapter 12

Anna Elizabeth "Klena" Hurlburt
–1956 School of Veterinary Medicine
Kansas State College

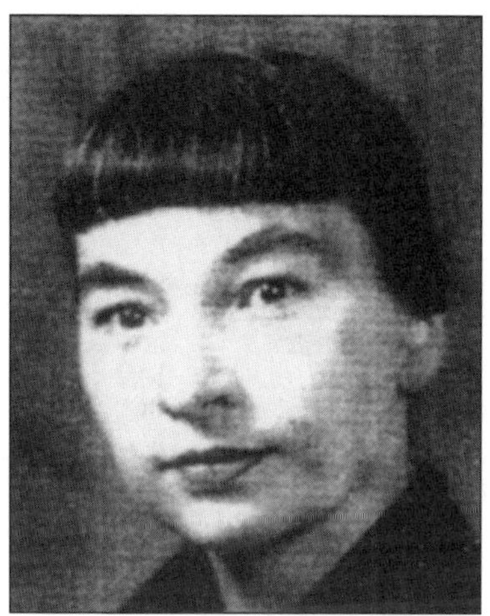

*A*nna Klena was the first child born to Emilia (Kmetz) Klena and her husband Martin F. Klena, in Newark, New Jersey. Anna and her elder sisters Amelia and Irene, (from a previous marriage) and younger brother Martin lived with their parents in Irvington, New Jersey. Anna and her bother Martin, attended Chancellor Avenue Elementary School, and Irvington High School.

Anna from a young age had a great love for animals, always surrounded by cats, dogs and horses. Anna at age three after visiting her grandfather's farm came home and announced that she was going to be a *horse vet*!

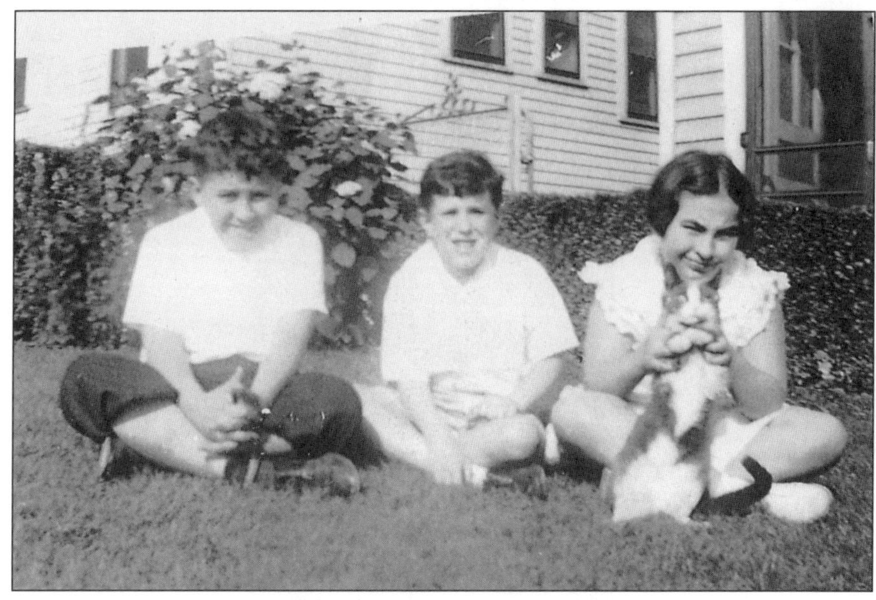

Anna with brother Marty, Cousin Louis and cats

She also had a passion for music which eventually was a big help when she applied to veterinary school.

Anna was an excellent student, and played in the high school band and orchestra. She worked in a deli after school to pay for music lessons. Anna became a percussionist and was proficient in playing the xylophone. She attended percussion lessons under the watchful eye of renowned percussionist Billy Dorn.

Her passion for music earned Anna a summer internship with the New York Philharmonic, a great honor. It was in 1944 that Anna received a musical scholarship to attend Cornell University, in New York.

Anna majored in music and minored in biological science at Cornell, with hope that she might attend veterinary school there. She enjoyed her classes and was privileged to be a student researcher to Rodger Tory Peterson, (American ornithologist, writer and illustrator) and Malcolm Miller (author of *Miller's Anatomy of the Dog*).

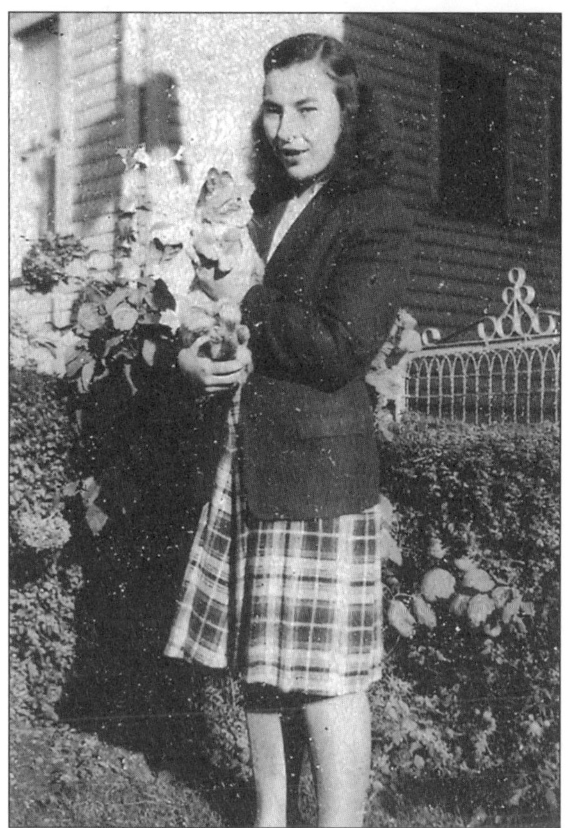

Anna with her cat "Alistair Duncan Malcolm
Montgomery Douglas Wallace Bruce Gordon Graham
Stewart, Lord McLennan," circa 1944

In 1948 she applied to the veterinary school at Cornell. Even though Cornell had admitted women to their veterinary curriculum in the past, Anna was turned down. The men were returning from World War Two, sadly denying Anna a place. Anna did not take kindly to this and challenged the admissions committee. Dr. Phyllis Larsen, 'KSC 1947, who was working in the Department of the Veterinary Experiment Station, (US Bureau of Animal Industry at Cornell University), remembers Anna telling her about her interview with the admissions committee. "It was a certain gentleman on the said committee, who mentioned that he felt because of Anna's short stature, he questioned if she were able to take care of farm animals of which she was interested in doing!" Anna who worked at one of the Cornell farms challenged the gentleman to join her in hefting sacks of grain and bales of hay! Maybe assertiveness was the reason Annie did not find favor with the admissions committee!"

Anna did not give in, and after her graduation from Cornell, went on a quest to find a veterinary school that would accept her.

Kansas State College graciously told her she would be accepted if she were to establish residency in Kansas. Anna moved to Atchison, Kansas, where she accepted a position as high school music teacher.

The following year in 1949, Anna had never been happier than when she was finally accepted into Kansas State College, School of Veterinary Medicine!

Anna was paired with a young man John "Jack" Hurlburt, for a lab partner. John was not pleased with having a 'feisty girl,' especially an eastern one, as his classmate. They were paired on many occasions and so he had to live with it!

Anna, who was nicknamed 'Annie' and 'Lena' in veterinary school, did exceptionally well in her classes. She was well liked and helped struggling classmates so that they might pass.

Possibly, through alphabetical pairing, John and Anna were thrown together many times, and started to enjoy each others company! It was not unusual to see them together off campus. Their interests in music, walking, bird watching, art, literature and dancing kept them close.

John introduced Anna to ranching and even went as far as buying a pair of 'Hyer' cowboy boots for her birthday. She loved to ride horses and was quite an accomplished horsewoman!

John and Anna were united in marriage on 30 December, 1950.

The next few years were a busy time for the Hurlburt's. Anna kept up her music skills by playing in the Kansas State College Band. She dropped out of veterinary school in the spring of 1952, to give birth to their firstborn, a son Daniel, born February 27.

John graduated from veterinary school in 1953, the family moved from Manhattan to Old Randolph, where he practiced for a few years.

Anna assisted John in their practice, and gave music lessons. It was after one more move and giving birth to their second child, a baby girl Kathleen, born 20 May, 1955, that Annie returned to veterinary school. She graduated with the class of 1956, alongside 64 men.

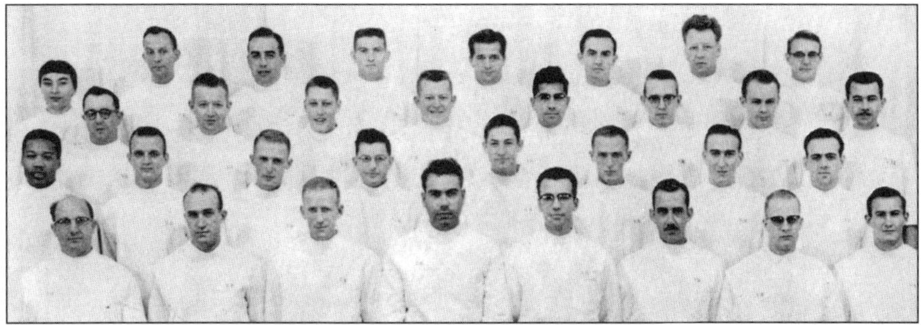

Anna with classmmates, circa 1956

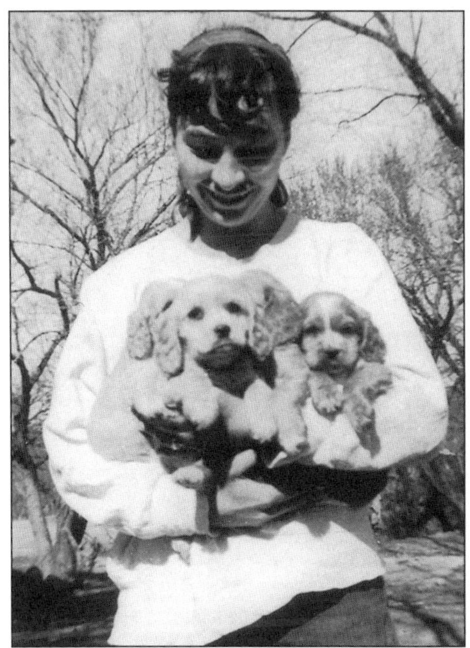

Anna with her cocker spaniel pups, Riley, KS

Anna, with her husband John, built and operated a practice in Riley, Kansas. Whilst Anna took care of the smaller animals, John took care of the large animals.

Anna juggled her time between caring for animals and her family. She enjoyed community events and became active in community affairs. She was active in her church and saw that her children attended Sunday school, of which she became the choir leader. Anna loved her garden and enjoyed finding new plants for her family's yard.

Anna was known for her kind and compassionate caring ways in the community. Her husband John remembers the day before Christmas one year, when a person brought a pregnant dog to Anna to be euthanized. Anna could not do this, especially the day before Christmas, so she took the dog in and took care of it until it whelped. She found homes for the puppies and gave the mother dog to a young boy whose parents had divorced.

The Hurlburt family enjoyed animals, having dogs, horses, rabbits, pigeons, poultry and Siamese cats of which Anna raised.

Anna and John were blessed on January 1, 1957, with a third child, a baby girl Mary, and again August 24, 1960, with baby boy James.

Anna enjoyed teaching young people to take care of animals. She became a 4-H leader, becoming active at all levels in the county and state. She was proud to have each of her children show cattle and horses in 4-H. Anna made sure each child played an instrument; she helped each one so that they became proficient and good musicians.

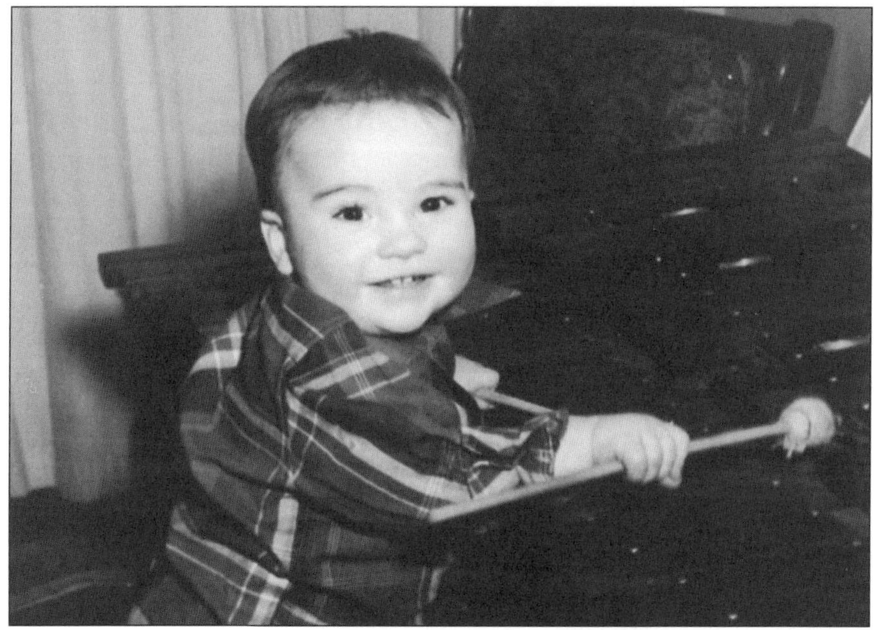

Daniel with Anna's xylophone, February 1953

Tragically on the evening of July 11, 1967, John and Anna's firstborn Daniel was fatally wounded by accidental gunfire, leaving a tremendous void in their lives. The Hurlburt family went on with their lives as best they could.

Anna was privileged to put her teaching skills to further use in 1976, when she joined the faculty at KSU College of Veterinary Medicine as an instructor in the Anatomy and Physiology Department.

Anna was a good teacher, her kind manner always helping discouraged students to regain composure and move on. She in turn was enjoyed, and remembered fondly by old students.

Anna was honored in 1977, as a recipient of the Humane Kindness Award. She was lauded for kindness not only to animals, but also to people. Annie enjoyed taking care of wildlife, and with the help of Dr. Kruckenburg, and Dr. West, at the Dykstra hospital, at Kansas State University, many hawks, ducks, owls and songbirds were returned to the wild.

It was in 1978, that Anna was diagnosed with cancer. She felt that teaching was 'good medicine' for her, and taught until a month before she passed away on the June 3, 1979, at her home.

Anna lived a short life, but a full one. She was dedicated to veterinary medicine and all that it involved. At the time of her death she was working on her PhD.

She was a fine teacher and veterinarian!

A plaque to commemorate Anna's outstanding service to youth in 4-H, hangs at the building named after her 'Hurlburt Hall,' at the fairgrounds at Cico Park, in Manhattan, Kansas.

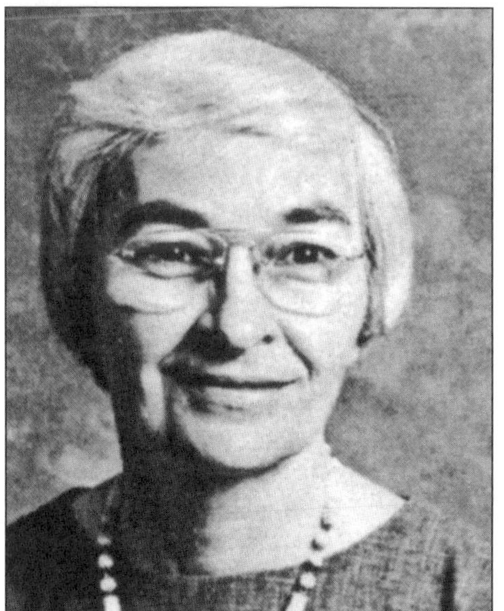

Dr. Anna Hurlburt, circa 1978

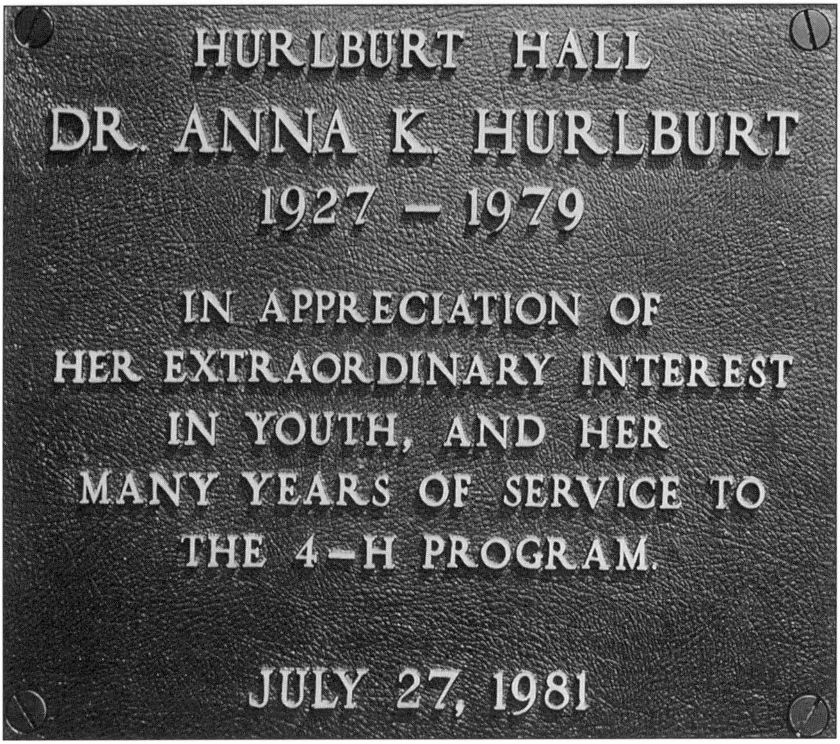

HURLBURT HALL
DR. ANNA K. HURLBURT
1927 — 1979

IN APPRECIATION OF
HER EXTRAORDINARY INTEREST
IN YOUTH, AND HER
MANY YEARS OF SERVICE TO
THE 4-H PROGRAM.

JULY 27, 1981

Anna Elizabeth "Klena" Hurlburt
Chronology

1918: 27 June, born Irvington, New Jersey

1933: Attended Chancellor Avenue Elementary School

1944: June, graduated Irvington High School, New Jersey
November
Given a musical scholarship to attend Cornell University

1948: Graduated from Cornell University, with B. S. in music and
biological science
Moved to Kansas, to establish residency.

1949: 12 September, admitted to the professional curriculum at Kansas
State College, School of Veterinary Medicine.

1950: 30 December, married John H. Hurlburt

1952: 27 February, Birth of first child, son Daniel John.

1955: 20 May, Birth of a daughter Kathleen Jane.

1956: 27 May, graduated from the professional curriculum at Kansas State
College, School of Veterinary Medicine.
Practiced with husband John (Jack).

1957 : 2 January, birth of third child, daughter Mary.

1960 : 24 August, birth of fourth child, son James.

1967 : 11 July, Son Daniel died in tragic accident.

*1976–
1979* : Joined the faculty at Kansas State College School of Veterinary Medicine as instructor in the Anatomy and Physiology Department.

1977 : April, Recipient of the Riley County Humane Society Kindness Award. Received 4-H award for service to the youth of the area.

1979 : 3 June, died at her home in Riley, Kansas, age 51.

1981 : Livestock show facilty at Cico Park Fairgrounds, Manhattan, Kansas, named "Hurlburt Hall."

They say we should not live in the past and I have no reason to do so because I am a practicing veterinary surgeon, still enjoying life. But to me, my past is a sweet and safe place to be...

—James Herriot M.R.C.V.S.

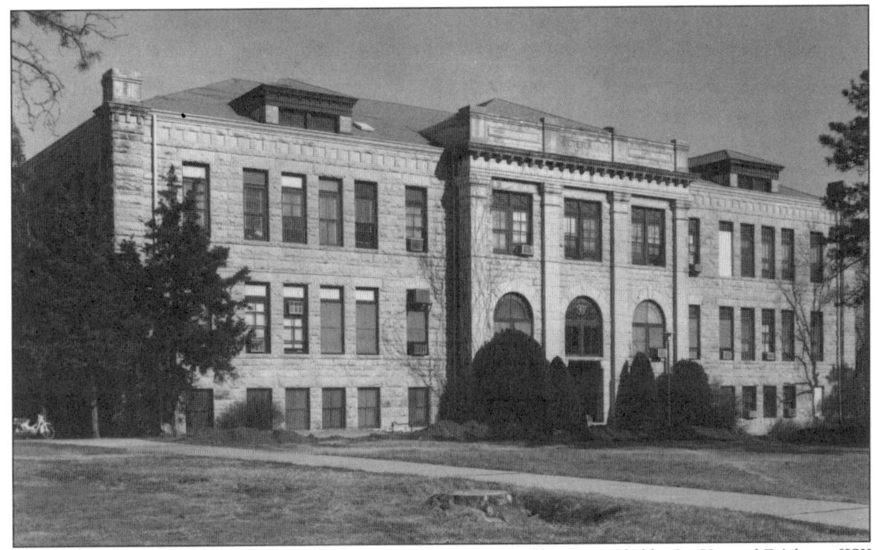

The Veterinary Building was built in 1907-08 and named Leasure Hall in 1969 for Dr. E. E. Leasure, who joined the faculty in 1926 and served as Dean of the College from 1948-64.

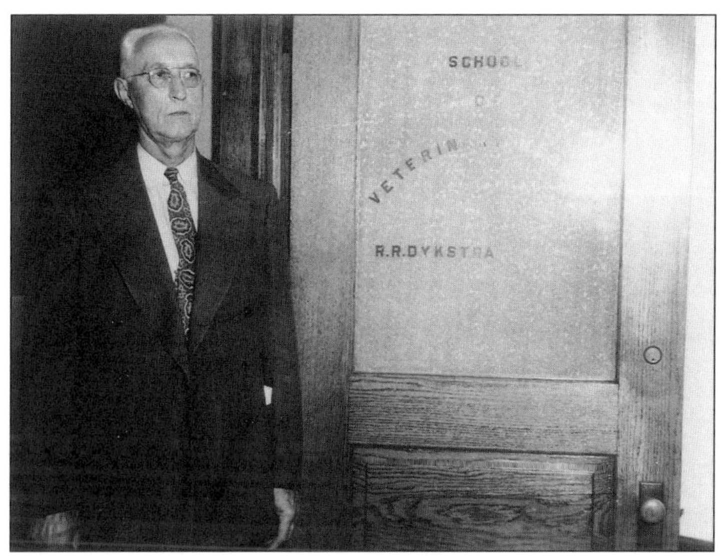

r. Ralph Dykstra joined the faculty in 1911. He became Dean of the Veterinary Division, a position he held until 1948. He was succeeded by Dr. E.E. Leasure.

1930–1931

Status	R	N
Total	43.00	60.00
Incidental	25.00	37.00
Matriculation	10.00	15.00
Health	3.00	3.00
Activity	5.00	5.00

R= Resident; N = Non-Resident
Matriculation fee is paid once only
Payment of health and activity fees is optional for graduate students

Books range from $8.50–31.30 for the first semester (depending on curricula)
Board in clubs and boarding houses averages $5.00–7.00/week
Rooms cost from $10.00–$15.00/month (higher priced rooms include light, heat and bath)

1935–1936

Status	R	N
Total	37.75	63.50
Incidental	18.75	37.00
Matriculation	7.50	15.00
Health	4.00	4.00
Activity	7.50	7.50

R= Resident; N = Non-Resident
Matriculation fee is paid once only
Payment of health and activity fees is optional for graduate students

Books range from $13.50–32.35 for the first semester (depending on curricula)
Board in clubs and boarding houses averages $3.00/week
Rooms cost from $6.00–8.00/month each (for a two person room)

1940–1941

Status	R	N
Total	47.50	107.50
Incidental	25.00	75.00
Matriculation	10.00	20.00
Health	5.00	5.00
Activity	7.50	7.50

R= Resident; N = Non-Resident
Matriculation fee is paid once only
Payment of health and activity fees is optional for graduate students

Books cost approx. $20 for the first semester (freshman year)
Board in clubs and boarding houses averages $4.00/week
Rooms cost from $7.00–9.00/month each (for a two person room)

1944–1946

Status	R	N
Total	55.00	115.00
Incidental	25.00	75.00
Matriculation	10.00	20.00
Health	7.50	7.50
Activity	7.50	7.50
Union	5.00	5.00

R= Resident; N = Non-Resident
Matriculation fee is paid once only
Payment of health and activity fees is optional for graduate students

Books cost approx. $20.00 for the first semester (freshman year)
Board in clubs and boarding houses averages $6.00/week
Rooms cost from $9.00–12.00/month each (for a two person room)

1950–1951

Status	R	RV	N	NV
Total	72.50	82.50	132.50	142.50
Incidental	50.00	60.00	100.00	110.00
Matriculation	10.00	10.00	20.00	20.00
Health	7.50	7.50	7.50	7.50
Union	5.00	5.00	5.00	5.00

R= Resident; N = Non-Resident; V = Vet Med
Matriculation fee is paid once only

Books cost approx. $30.00 for the first semester (freshman year)

1955–1956

Status	R	RV	N	NV
Total	90.00	100.00	165.00	175.00
Incidental	56.00	66.00	131.00	141.00
Health	10.00	10.00	10.00	10.00
Union	7.50	7.50	7.50	7.50
Activity	16.50	16.50	16.50	16.50

R= Resident; N = Non-Resident; V = Vet Med
Matriculation fee is paid once only

Books cost approx. $30.00 for the first semester (freshman year)

Information provided by Hale Library, KSU

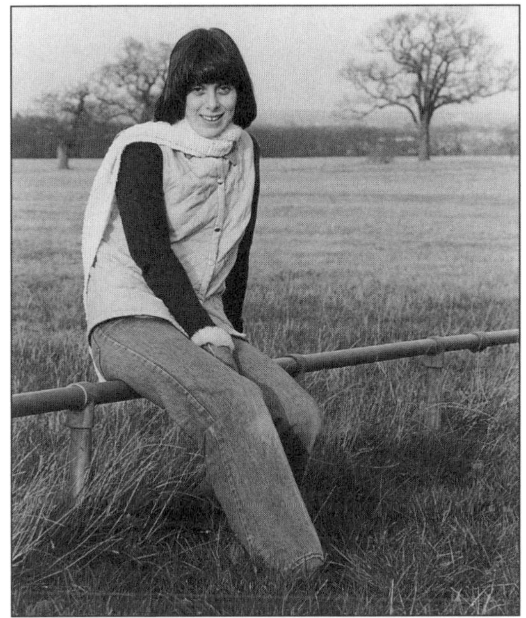

Photo by Paul M. Stevens

*L*esley Ann Gentry has spent over 25 years working in veterinary practice. Born and raised in England, she currently resides in Beloit, Kansas with her husband Robert, daughter Jamie and son Paul. Together, the family operates a veterinary practice in Beloit.

Lesley has had articles published in "Cats Magazine," "Cat World," "Mule Magazine," and "US Veterinarian 2005," as well as several other small articles. She enjoys writing and has been a member of the Kansas Authors Club for a number of years. "The Lady is a Veterinarian," is her first book.

Having a great interest in history and veterinary medicine, Lesley felt compelled to write an account of the pioneer women who graduated from Kansas State College School of Veterinary Medicine. She believes that they are an important part of history and should not be forgotten. After several years of research, she is proud to honor these 'ladies' with "The Lady Is A Veterinarian."